SKIN HEALTH

Surgical Alternatives to Healthy Skin
Anti-Aging and Scar Revision

UPDATED AND REVISED

Danné Montague-King

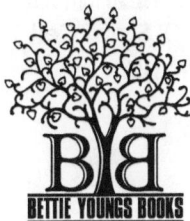

BETTIE YOUNGS BOOKS

www.BettieYoungsBooks.com

Cover Design: Erin Lup at DMK Marketing,
and Beau Kimbrel, Kimbrel Designs
Text Design: Beau Kimbrel, Kimbrel Designs

BETTIE YOUNGS BOOK PUBLISHERS, Inc.,
www.Bettie Youngs Books.com.

If you are unable to order this book from your local bookseller, or online, or Ingram Book Group, order direct from the publisher: info@BettieYoungsBooks.com

Print ISBN: 978-1-940784-66-3
Digital ISBN: 978-1-940784-67-0

Library of Congress Control Number Available upon Request.

1. Skin Health. 2. Alternatives to Surgery. 3. Skin Procedures.
4. DMK International. 5. Diet and Nutrition. 6. Vitamins.
7. Acne. 8. Skin Diseases. 9. Stem Cell Therapy. 10. Melanin.
11. Enzyme Therapy. 12. Aging.

10 9 8 7 6 5

OTHER BOOKS BY THE AUTHOR

The Maybelline Prince

TABLE OF CONTENTS

ABOUT DANNÉ MONTAGUE-KING

Skin treatment pioneer Danné Montague-King discusses his 50 years of research pioneering a skin revision methodology. Inspired to self-treat his own severe bouts of acne, Danné soon realized that human cells will not accept that which is either nonessential to their natural make up or is not recognized as workable fuel. It was his first major discovery.

"It has long been my contention that the cells of the body are not programmed to die easily. They are programmed to stay alive if possible, and can, given the right maintenance and environmental surroundings," says the skin-care industry giant. *"I quickly saw how other skin conditions such as acne or aging affect skin problems; it's exciting to see just how much we really can effect. My concept is based upon the principles of the skin's biochemistry: Remove, Rebuild, Protect, Maintain."*

Mr. Montague-King began his work teaching skin revision in beauty schools around Chicago in the 80's, then left Chicago for California to host a television series called *Skin Deep*. He then continued his research in skin care, addressing it in term of functionality and hormonal fluctuation (for example, acne starting in the hypothalamus gland and cortisol levels contributed to many skin problems).

Ever an innovator, Danné was the first scientist in his field to recognize the power of enzymes in skin treatment, such as its ability to hydrolyze dead skin cells—and not enzymes in the products, but the idea of stimulating the many enzymes already in the skin and body that orchestrate everything. "It's really very easy to understand," says Danné. *"The human body is a bag of fluids containing a few chemicals that are orchestrated by enzymes and held together with electromagnetic waves."*

The frontrunner of the worldwide movement known as Skin Revision, Mr. Montague-King's "Remove–Rebuild–Protect–Maintain" system revolutionized the way skincare is approached the world over. As an expert in medical chemistry and biophysics, Danné and his team at DMK International have pioneered many of the current treatments popular today. He formulated a topical analgesic based on cryotherapy that he called BIOFREEZE™—which is now one of the most famous products in the world. Selling out his interest and formula for

BIOFREEZE™, Danné then worked with the world's leading physicians and surgeons in an effort to elevate the importance of proper pre- and post-operative skin revision protocol, surgical alternatives, scar revision, and skin health maintenance, looking for long term results.

Known as the ultimate therapist's and aesthetic medical practitioner's advocate, Danné remains a tireless educator and researcher. He travels the world conducting lectures to professionals and consumers alike, often participating in hands-on training. As one of the most published aesthetic journalists in the world, Danné Montague-King is a regular contributor to many of the most important professional magazines; his articles have been published in 20 languages worldwide.

His exhaustive research on darker toned skins in South Africa (which sparked the movement against "Whiter is better" which was better known as "Don't Mess With My Skin" and supported by South African skin activist Najma Kahn), won him a "Democracy Means Freedom to Choose" accommodation from Prince Mangosuthu Butjelaizi, Zula King (currently Prime Minister) in June, 2019.

Danné Montague-King is a name synonymous with world-class skin revision and products available in over twenty countries. He is also the creator of several "firsts" that globally have helped others have a better quality of life. These include BIOFREEZE™, DMK Foundations of Skin, DMK Skin Revision, and DEEP FREEZE. Danné is the recipient of numerous awards, including the prestigious Global Human Rights Ambassador Award by the Harvey Milk Foundation.

In 2016, he was named their Global Ambassador. Danné's book, *"The Maybelline Prince,"* a memoir about his life and times as a business partner with Evelyn F. Williams, sister-in-law of Tom Lyle Williams, Founder of the iconic Maybelline company, is published by Bettie Youngs Book Publishers, Inc. (www.BettieYoungsBooks.com) and is available world-wide.

Danné Montague-King
www.DMKCosmetics.com
www.DannéMKing.com

PREFACE

As far back as I can remember, even as a boy with a kid's chemistry set and later as a teenage acne victim, I was always curious about how things in the body really worked.

Today, at age 75, I am still that little boy, challenging everything that does not sound logical—especially things advertised as "the best" or "a miracle." Our own bodies are the miracle, an organic computer capable of healing and renewing itself over and over in a lifetime, so I'm naturally suspect when products are advertised to do things I doubt is true. This book is largely about looking at some real facts, versus myths, in that regard.

I do practice what I preach. Textbooks, no matter how in-depth, become dated and change from time to time. I use my eyes, sense of logic and often my gut instinct, to explore and discover ways and means to care for, as well as alleviate the suffering, of my clients.

It has been a wonderful and fantastic journey for over 50 years of seeing and often personally experiencing old and new technology; I am my first and foremost guinea pig on every new idea I come up with!

I have never found just one product, machine or medical innovation, to reinstate youth or healthy skin. It really does take teamwork on behalf of the client and the professional practitioner, to evoke results in skin anomalies. At times, it can take many, many treatments using combinations of modalities. But the way we look is a personal feeling, not just an outake feature. Beautiful skin, healthy skin, will always be an ideal. I'm hoping this book and the years I've spent perfecting skincare methods is helpful to you. That is truly my goal.

Danné Montague-King, Author

DMK

Danné Montague-King®

10420 Pioneer Blvd.
Santa Fe Springs, CA 90670, USA
888-DANNE-4-U or 888-326-6348
www.DannéMKing.com

1

Aging: How You Can Look and Feel Better, Longer

In Singapore, years ago, there was a huge photo of me on the side of a tall building (trying to look like a GQ male model!).

The caption under the photo read: *"Age Does Not Matter, Looking Good Does."* I'll admit that it is a quote I made!

My only defense is akin to the Chinese Philosopher's statement, *"We are born, and we die: whatever happens in between is up to us."* The truth is, like most all of us, I enjoy looking and feeling good. That said, confidence on the "outside" can and does influence our inner well-being. Research shows that the way we feel, our basic happiness and contentment with our lives, contributes to our overall health and well-being. The concept of "more than skin deep" is real.

No matter how we may feel inside, we have the tools to maintain the outside and even improve on the original model! When we look and feel our very best, our confidence soars and we better summon up the determination to face life with gusto and joy! I call this "confidence from outside in!"

Healthy skin, a proper weight, a healthy sense of self and dressed nicely for one's body type, are all part of the package called "looking good."

The pull of gravity, too much exposure to the sun, a stress-filled life, as well as hormone flux, show up in the skin. But we can do something about it. The first thing we can do is to take better care of ourselves. Year by year, lifestyle, stress, nutrition, drug and alcohol use, take their toll.

I enjoy feeling good, and, looking good. I think we can do that at any age, if we are vigilant in the self-care areas.

Maintaining a look of health and vibrancy is possible. And as I said, it has payoffs.

Looking Good: Confidence from the Outside In

Laser treatments, surgical procedures, BOTOX® and fillers, while they can help, they are temporary fixes and not the answer to long term skin-care health. Healthy skin responds to all these high-tech modalities much better than skin that has been damaged and neglected. A person with badly sun damaged skin and a coarse texture reddened by transepidermal water loss, is NOT going to look 20 years younger with BOTOX® and a few fillers.

On the other hand, a person with skin that has consistently shed its redundant cuticle, has a healthy immune system and has hydrated his or her body appropriately, is more likely to have healthy skin, and as such, that person's skin can better bounce back time and again by moderate (versus aggressive) procedures. In short, that person is likely to look better longer. This person is more likely to look 20 years younger with these marvelous medical tweaks available today.

Who knows what it can be in the future: we are constantly looking to find better ways to treat the skin. That said, it will still be concept, as opposed to ingredients, that will rule the day. There are only so many mechanical ways one can treat the skin, only so many actions that can influence the cells and the vascular systems. Delivery is the most important factor (which by the way, does not always require penetrating the skin).

NANO technology is promising but we're light years away from SAFE NANOTECH for skin care. Currently NANO TECH scientists can compound delivery systems with tiny molecules that can reach the dermis, like a topically applied injection. But what then? What happens when these miniscule ingredients start piling up and then enter the body systemically? How does the body deal with this over time? And at what point will we know if something that is perfectly safe for the epidermis to handle, will be equally safe lodged in the kidneys, liver or vesicles to the heart?

Fortunately, there are labs that can gauge the size of the molecules and even the shape, so that there will be a control and monitoring factor. I'm extremely interested in where all this will lead us in the years ahead, which is why I love this area of "looking and feeling good."

Skincare (or skin revision, as I prefer to call it) is a most exciting field—one we're just now beginning to explore seriously.

2

The FDA's Hysteria and the Kitchen Chemist

After 50 years in the industry, I've seen everything come and go and then come back again. What irritates me most, is the hype and hysteria that surrounds an alleged new "miracle" ingredient. Once it was Matrixyl 2000, the so-called "nano spheres" (basically only micro spheres; it's unlikely we will never see real nano-size anything in the skincare, skin revision industry). Vitamin C has had many "big days," and many hurrahs, and has seen its fair share of competition over who offered it in its best form.

Since the 60s, I had been using plain old ascorbyl palmitate for the fibroblast cells in the skin to get faster collagen proliferation and because it is highly unstable. It is the strongest form of any co-enzyme. The word "unstable" to a chemist merely means any ingredient that denatures quickly when exposed to oxygen. When we stabilize a vitamin, we modify it from its strongest to a lower active power. I would surround my stable palmitate with three to four stabilized ascorbic acids, thus extending its life a little longer.

In between one of the "C crazes," the days of "Acid Reign" had everyone touting products containing alpha hydroxy acids (AHAs), disregarding whether daily use was good for the skin (it is not). This fad died out when microdermabrasion became popular. Then along came Retinol and all of vitamin A derivatives, followed by peptides (very weak little amino acids, not a primary treatment).

Currently we are in various stages of "injection crazed" with micro needling allowing beauty therapists to pretend they are doctors! Ironically, we have been doing all those things collectively for many, many years. All of this led to internet bloggers who started talking about ingredients, each spouting off pseudo-science on what is good, what is not, how much it takes, or what works best in the skin, and so on.

When I began the journey in this field decades ago, cosmetic ingredients were very simple and basic. The FDA was not looming over everything as it is nowadays. If we listed something as "safe" in the CTFA library, basically we could make anything we wanted. I was a "kitchen chemist" back then, cutting my early teeth since age 12 on Gilbert Chemistry sets. Ultimately my goal was to get rid of my own acne at age seventeen by almost fevered forays into the world of plants and herbs, imagining I was some sort of alchemist or "magic man." In those days, not being able to afford expensive extracts, I had to depend upon maceration (mine) of herbs (cold soak method) to get the action I thought the body would respond to. To this day my company, DMK International, produce many of our own raw materials in this time consuming, but predictable, manner.

Nowadays, raw material companies practically beg me to tour their premises—including Research and Development areas—and send out slick portfolios of their products, including MSDS sheets, the tech support. Their products have magical names such as Induchem's wonderful "Neodermyl" ingredient. Some time back, I sat in an audience of aestheticians listening to a self-proclaimed chemist regaling us with "miracle ingredients to come," touting Neodermyl as being available sometime in two or three years and we were to all "watch for it!" I had to laugh; my company had been using it for two years!

In my 50-years of being in the skin-health, skin revision field, I have seen everything come and go—and come back around again. Now 75, I have a more relaxed view of things that previously would make me livid with the outright fraud of it all. I have now been on the side of the practitioner, Doctor and therapist, and try to teach CONCEPT, as opposed to INGREDIENT.

Products are only tools to implement a concept. Yes, the best and most bioactive ingredients are important, but concept— which is a philosophy of logical science—is what purveyors of aesthetics should think about first. I always view the body as an organic computer, capable of repairing itself almost indefinitely—if given the right environment and daily support. We all must brush our teeth. We don't get up in the morning excited about brushing our teeth; we do it automatically or our breath will knock people over and our teeth will rot and fall out of our heads!

Our skin deserves no less consideration. Everything we do for our skin should rely on a simple, four-tiered concept:

- Remove (remove the dead cell build up);

- Rebuild (offer the living skin cells "food" that they recognize which will enable them to stay alive for as long as possible);

- Protect (bar free radicals and other environmental damage from attacking and destroying the living skin cells); and,

- Maintain (keeping all the above operating with full energy daily).

The final caution regarding ingredients, is to ask:

- What is the source? Many famous bioactive ingredients are grown in substandard soil or in countries that have little regulatory laws that insure the safety of their farms and botanical products.

- How are the ingredients processed? Being processed at a lab is vital since many ingredients denature when exposed to excessive heat.

- What is the delivery method of the ingredient and its percentage? If the base formula of the product does not go INTO the epidermis, and it's at a very low percent, the product is nearly useless (and a waste of money), no matter how popular the ingredient may be in the public marketplace.

I always view the body as an organic computer, capable of repairing itself almost indefinitely—if given the right environment and daily support.

3

Acne Vulgaris: Causes and Treatments

The press often says that I became involved in the skin—health business because of my own terrible bout with teenage acne. This is true in part; I remember everything about that time in the 1950s as if it were yesterday. I was the eldest child in an affluent and social family, and from birth to around age 12, I was always complimented on what a "pretty boy" I was! So naturally, I accepted and viewed myself as nice looking!

Suddenly "Acne Vulgaris" reared its ugly head and the nice looking boy had vanished, replaced by a reclusive and miserable youth who always put his head down when a photo was taken.

One of the nicknames given by my peer group during that time was "pizza face!" Hence, I totally understand what a lot of youth go through. I have devoted a great many years combating this scourge with methods that were originally thought to be unusual, but over time, have proven very effective.

The Role of Stress

When I was a teenager in the 1950s there was a popular over-the-counter product called "Clearasil," a sort of pinkish-beige tinted chalky creme, allegedly supposed to dry out acne and pimples. However, I had other uses for the product. I loathed appearing at school bristling with pustules, so I covered my entire face with this salve, a make-up base, to cover the offensive "pizza face" look. Unfortunately, the product really did dry out the skin and would crack with facial movements, hence I refrained from smiling at all, earning me an even worse title, "The Death-Mask Kid!"

It all sounds funny now, but to a young person suffering from peer group pressure, an acne condition is far from amusing. I recall in 1994 when I was appearing on the Dublin chat show "Kenny Live" (Ireland's answer to Oprah Winfrey and Geraldo Rivera) and my topic was acne conditions. The preceding evening the newspaper headlined the story about a youth who committed suicide because of his severe acne and lack of money to treat it!

There really is a hopeless and unclean feeling when you are an acne victim. You feel especially vulnerable to the opposite sex in those growing years, positive that every girl (or boy) recoils in disgust when you enter the room. Imagine the fear of being up close to others; it's a really shame-filled feeling.

I am determined to help others not have to experience that.

At seventeen, I decided to do something about my condition. My parents trotted me to every dermatologist in town, with no success (the treatments in those days were archaic, as even in some cases today). I felt that using Ivory soap twice a day, along with astringents, was the wrong approach.

I Was Determined to "Cure" my Acne

Being a kitchen-chemist in those early years, I knew about acids and alkalis. A medical friend taught me about the pH of the skin and its slightly acid sebaceous oil. I also knew that the base of all bars of soaps contained alkaloids. After all, the first soaps were made from ash and fats. It occurred to me that the alkaloids in commercial bars of soap, no matter how pure or botanical the oils used in manufacturing them, would turn the acid oil in my skin into pre-deposited fats, as well. In other words, it would create tiny plugs of soap, or wax, in my pores!

Reading up on American Indian lore and methods about how the ancients used to clean their bodies, I discovered the powers of natural saponin obtained from certain tree barks. I stripped some of these barks from trees, soaked them in water and pounded the inside cellulose into a pulp. I then filtered this pulp into a bottle, added a little powdered ascorbic acid as a preservative, and started using this odd smelling concoction to cleanse my face.

I also started whipping up odd masks made from oatmeal, tomato, okra, and wheatgerm. I made a crude creme with sodium alginate, olive oil, and again, vitamin C. This seemed to hold water in my skin without being greasy, as were conventional moisture cremes of the day. I also altered my diet and refused greasy chips, hamburgers and fatty foods. I increased water consumption instead of soft drinks and went on a work-out program for two hours a day!

I was determined to be as handsome and as popular as the blemish-free guys at school.

As I looked in the mirror over the months of my 17th year, I could see changes happening. As it did, the stress and fears of being ugly started to vanish. Confidence soared!

When I turned 18, girls were approaching me in the halls. I was invited to gatherings and parties, as much for my caustic wit as my looks, but at least I was no longer unafraid to attend and no longer sat the shadowy corners, as I had before. I had come into the light at last!

This experience taught me that things CAN be changed. Years later as we learned more and more about the condition of acne, the changes of my youth suddenly had a reason behind them. As a scientist I always want to know why something works, not just that it does.

Causes of Acne

There are many varieties of acne. It takes specific training to recognize and diagnose each basic category or combinations of categories, but stress is hands-down a major player in many acne conditions. There are other contributing factors as well, including lifestyle, climate, diet, heredity and others, but stress tops the list as a real menace.

There is a gland at the top of the head called the Hypothalamus. Think of it as sort of a radio antenna that receives all signals of stress confronting the human body. The signal is relayed from the gland to the Pituitary (the master gland) located further down at the base of the skull.

The Pituitary gland, receiving this message of stress, picks up his telephone and repeats the message to Mr. and Mrs. Adrenal glands, who in their excitement wake up Tommy Testosterone! Now Tommy, although a male hormone, also has relatives living in all female bodies. All the Testosterone folks get together and shout at the Hair Follicle Family to not only increase the hair population, but to pump more sebaceous oil onto the skin.

This aggressive relay of messages is all due to stress, which falls into several categories, including:

- Subliminal stress (adult acne). The person does not know why he or she is stressed but it subconsciously exists and may well require counseling or even psychiatric assistance, as well as treatment of the skin, to overcome.

- <u>Hormonal stress</u> (passive). Females go through several hormonal changes throughout their lifetime. They can break out in acne during any one of these times, or all of them. Many women for instance, have peaches and creme complexion until they have their first baby—then it's "Pizza Face" time! After going through menopause, some women may suddenly develop acne after years of perfect skin. Men will have some hormonal changes as well, but usually just during puberty. Sometimes there may be a deeply hidden pathological reason for severe hormonal changes which require the services of a competent endocrinologist before advanced skin treatment is undertaken.

- <u>Job-related Stress.</u> This type of stress can create serious trauma to the adrenal glands. It can be caused by an anxiety-laden work load, feelings of inadequacy within the job or position itself, conflicts with staff or management, threats of layoffs, being firing and so on. In other words, it's a person to person stress comparison.

- <u>Emotional Stress:</u> Feeling unworthy, "not being good enough," feelings of hopelessness, being trapped, and misunderstood, all keeping your mind stirred up and emotions in a tailspin.

- <u>Adolescence trauma, bullying, or extreme and unabated peer pressure.</u> A stress-filled existence in the early years can set psychological patterns of ill-fated coping that repeat themselves in adulthood, and keep the emotions stirred up and the body in a constant state of flux.

- <u>PC Skin:</u> Positive charged electromagnetic waves coming off a computer, when sitting in front of a computer for as much as eight hours a day, upsets the central nervous system and can result in rosacea like symptoms.

Managing the Imbalance that Leads to Acne

The question of course, is how to treat acne so as to relieve this condition. This depends on two things: the pH of ingredient (too alkaline being "bad") and the viscosity or molecular structure of the ingredient which determines whether it is fractioned enough to be water soluble and work WITH the skin secretions, rather than trying to replace them.

There are thousands of little openings in the skin with secretive functions. Anything heavier than these secretions will plug or clog the pores. Mineral oil is an example of a "bad" ingredient, but we have one plant-based salve formula for that. When applied to a hardened cystic-type pustule, it will hydrolyze away the infection inside the pustule within 24 hours. This application works on the principle of creating pseudo-heat within the pustule, plus the power of a very effective anti-bacterial stabilizer that destroys gram positive / negative bacteria.

Although it really is a matter of opinion and experience regarding good and bad ingredients, the important thing is that the skin must be decongested first, then the acid mantle restored to normal, and finally, the flow of sebaceous oil regulated. Basically, we are talking about the "remove" and "restore" process.

The macrophagic action of enzymes and the fact that they are nature's biological catalysts for all the skin's interactions, make enzyme treatments possibly the most superior dead skin cell removal system for acne skins. Alkaline Wash desquamates (exfoliates) keratin build-up that clogs the pores. Revitosin removes and rebuilds tissue that is compromised by cuneiform scars.

Alpha Hydroxy Acids and Benzoyl Peroxide

Several types of glycolic acid can irritate and ultimately re-inflame acne skins due to the "stripping" action of skin fluids (AHAs work off these fluids). However, a well-blended, multiple AHA formula in a low strength makes a wonderful removal system if applied to the skin as an "occlusion" masque under strips of cling film (such as Glad Wrap). This approach really breaks up those annoying hard-to-get-out milia and allows extraction with minimal scar causing pressure.

AHAs are not for home use on acne, despite the current

popularity of AHA products.

Playing Piano on the pH Scale is my descriptive way of naming treatments that rapidly change the pH of the skin to very low (acid) or very high (alkaline). These types of treatments are like fighting fire, yet can be very effective when used in conjunction with enzyme treatments. An acid formula will "harden" the dead and dying corneum very quickly and the brittle cells then sort of "pop off." An alkaline solution will soften the corneum, and any keratinized proteins on the skin, as well as hair. This is very good for folliculitis conditions.

Both styles of therapy must be carefully monitored, require advance training, and of course the client's normal pH must be restored at the conclusion of these types of treatment, each time they are performed.

Benzoyl Peroxide lotions and ointments have been around a long time. Benzoyl Peroxide products must be in a gel-base or water-soluble gel/creme base to be effective. Peroxide releases powerful oxygen into the skin which kills bacteria. The Benzoyl part of the molecule pulls the peroxide down into the pore or follicle where the Corynebacterium (C acnes) are located, killing them off very quickly. For countries where Benzoyl Peroxide is not allowed, we have many even more effective alternatives.

A Healthy Diet

In the treatment of acne, a healthy diet is essential and although chocolate and greasy foods are not the primary cause of acne, they do add to the situation. Many with acne also suffer from candida and have very alkaline systems.

Certain vitamins and supplements (vitamin C, Zinc) can help, but be careful to properly take the correct supplements and dosages. If you are unsure, check with a pharmacist or dermatologist.

There are many approaches to acne treatment, and of course some physicians feel that drug treatment is the only cure, while cosmetic treatment only cleans the skin. My experience has been that the cells of the skin respond to the chemistry that they recognize, indeed the very chemistry they are made of.

If a cell is receiving positive electromagnetic charges from the brain, the sodium surrounding the cell (also a positive ion) will be pulled into the cell itself and vital potassium inside the cell (negative ion) will be pulled out. The cell then goes into trauma and inflammation starts running amok. Infection enters the picture and the trauma spreads. You then have a diseased cell. On the other hand, if the electromagnetic charge from the brain is changed to a negative charge to the cell, the cell becomes re-polarized, and trauma disappears and the cell starts functioning normally.

SCAR REVISION AND ENZYME TREATMENTS

Many teenagers have superficial acne scars that appear purplish or red. This is a good age to undergo scar revision while the skin is in growing mode. Unlike "Ice Pick Scars" that require more intense methods of skin planning such as dermabrasion, laser treatment, or the Mon's Tissue Transplant method, teenage acne scars are often removed easily with enzyme treatments.

This type of treatment allows the newer, underlying skin cells to rebuild the surface appearance. Advanced training is required of the aesthetician, as these types of treatment may take from six weeks to as long as eight months, to show significant results. There will, however, always be results! More on this later.

4

Peels, Enzymes and Electromagnetic Waves

In the skin-care world, *peel* is a popular buzz word. There are many kinds of peels: bio-peel, phyto-peel, and chemi-peel, to name a few. The idea behind peeling comes originally from medical peels performed usually by a plastic surgeon (and at a high cost and can have an uncomfortable convalescence for the client).

These medical procedures normally involve a high percent of phenol acid, which is effective in completely removing the epidermis. The results are very good if performed under optimum conditions. They are also quite effective in removing fine wrinkles, hyperspotty pigmentation, and light acne scars. A new epidermis grows back in a few months looking permanently younger but sometimes faintly artificial. Darker toned skins are not the best candidates for this procedure due to keloid and depigmentation potentials.

The medical peel does not lift sagging skin as some "before" and "after" photos in advertisements would have you believe. Only surgery can totally excise sagging skin. Chemical peels are for wrinkle erasure only, many times done after a surgical face lift. Because of the enormous edema (swelling) caused by the peel process, some patients experience a fuller thus more youthfully contoured face for a few weeks—which probably gave birth to the lift claims. But after the edema subsides, the normal contours return without the wrinkles.

Bad effects following a peel usually are in the form of pronounced millia and the Peau de Orange or Orange Peel effects. This is enlarged pores which have been totally exposed by the peel. At this time the aestheticians can do vital work on the client as there is no old epidermis to penetrate. Using the right chemistry, chemistry the body recognizes, the aesthetician can obliterate large pores and tighten up skin considerably.

Peeling Isn't Enough

Personally, I am opposed to the term "peel." While I recognize the validity of the medical peel, newer methods bring about similar results as the medical peel without the lengthy convalescence and a have more natural appearance. The aesthetician may not be able to flash-burn off the old epidermis like the physician, but he or she can hydrolyze it off while encouraging the collagen fibrils in the skin to produce more rapidly. The result is skin that is progressively tighter, younger, and healthy. But, peeling isn't enough; applications to regenerate the skin must be employed simultaneously.

The word *hydrolyze* in this case means to turn dead cells into a weak base acid and get rid of them. As the skin is not really in definite layers (but rather a series of hills and valleys with cells pushing against old cells) exfoliation via scuffing pads, beauty grains, or almond and honey scrubs, are ineffective and ultimately damaging to the skin.

Among the worst of this methods offered is the crushed Pearl lotion—hyped with the idea that oriental women don't age (they do!); they've used this preparation for centuries. When you consider a pearl is formulated as a result of an oyster secreting vomit around a piece of sand to stop the irritation, you can draw your own conclusions as to the validity of this product!

When you hydrolyze dead keratin, you more quickly reach all the hills and valleys in the skin. Soon you have just the living cells left behind to work with. Your goal is to encourage their development and keep them alive a little bit longer, thus slowing age. When all the cells are cleaned out, gases, effluvia, and secretion-blocking debris start to disappear—and problems such as acne and dermatitis, vanish. You can readily see the improvements.

ENZYMES AND HYDROLYZATION

Enzyme action is another popular buzz phrase. With all the recent talk about enzymes, you'd think enzymes were invented only yesterday. In fact, no living organism on this planet, from the dawn of time, could exist without the catalytic cooperation of enzymes.

In skin treatments, enzymes can eat up to thirty five (35) times their weight in dead cell material. Containing little microorganisms, known as macrophages, enzymes can clean out all the paraplastic debris and gases in forty-five (45) minutes. Common enzymes like papaya or papain have been used for years, before intense research yielded more highly sophisticated groups of enzymic activity for skin treatment.

But enzymes do much more than eat up dead cells. They act as biological catalysts, speeding up chemical reactions in the skin, by increasing the frequency of molecular collisions, lowering the activation energy (amount of energy required for chemical reactions to take place), and properly orienting the colliding molecules where they are supposed to go. Once the dead cell layer is removed, further action in the production of new collagen and elastin fibers is highly accelerated. The result is tighter, firmer skin.

Human Collagen vs Animal Collagen

Human collagen production must not be confused with animal by-product collagen, which by the medical law of rejection is not accepted by the human body permanently, whether by injection or topical application. Common sense tells us that human and animal genetic blueprints are not the same. All our collagen is manufactured by the fibroblast cell, a factory-like cell that rather resembles a little octopus under a microscope. Set off by common vitamin C, amino acids such as Lysine and Proline are pushed into the first stage of producing tropocollagen (baby collagen) which makes a trip through the fibroblast factory, as though on a conveyor belt.

From time to time different nutrients are added, including certain carbohydrates, until the now mature collagen bursts through the wall of the fibroblast cell as full-blown collagen fibrils floating and winding their way through the base substance of the skin's cell structure. Looking a bit like cables or ropes, these collagen fibrils along with their sister cell, the elastin, are responsible for the lift or tightness in the skin.

Vitamin C is vital to collagen synthesis. I've used Vitamin C, both orally and topically, extensively over the last twenty-five years with clients and the results are excellent.

ELECTROMAGNETIC THERAPY

In my opinion, electromagnetic therapy will make all facial machines as we know them today, obsolete. The biological effects of electromagnetic energy have been known since the turn of the century when famed French scientist D'Arsonval noted effects completely distinct from those due to any local heating—therefore improved circulation of tissue.

In the medical field, short pulses of high frequency EME (Electromagnetic Energy) followed by relatively long intervals, have shown two principle properties: reduction of inflammation of stress, and acceleration of wound-healing following an operation or injury.

Evidence shows that these effects take place within the cell and probably at the level of protein macromolecules, which are the prime constituent of all living matter. The EME waves repolarizes protein molecules and help restore the normal trans-membrane potential. Low intensity energy between 150-250 Mhz—the electrical resonance range of protein—is an exclusive adaptation of Electromagnetic Energy via several body contact antennas traditionally designed for the skin therapist working in a state-of-the-art facility. Former devices were available to medical personnel only, and was cost prohibitive to the average person.

Not only does electromagnetic energy speed up collagen production in tissue, but when used in conjunction with plant enzymes and pure botanical skin treatment formulas, accelerate the actions of these formulas 100 times faster. There is evidence that electromagnetic waves influence the matrix, or ground substance. All living cells float in this, relieving pressure on new cells and allowing them to develop faster.

Sir Thomas C. Smith, MD, one of the world's leading experts on cell rejuvenation, when confronted with EMR apparatus in 1988, stated, *"These devices immediately remove stress from the patients when applied to the body. If that is all that happened it would be enough!"*

Doctor Smith was referring to the fact that research has shown stress to be a major cause of rapid aging and acne conditions—by setting off undesirable chemical reactions throughout the body.

Sagging face and body skin; acne; sun-damaged skins; couperose skin; hyperpigmentation and cellulite, are but a few examples of skin treatments using EMW modalities along with topical treatment.

5

Skin Tone is a Matter of Melanin

Melanin is a dark brown to black pigment in the hair, skin, and iris of the eye, in both people and animals. Its purpose is to protect the skin when exposed to sunlight.

In the 1990s I was spending a great deal of time in Hong Kong, Singapore, Malaysia, and Thailand, teaching about skin revision. While there, I paid close attention to the emphasis each country placed on health—such as nutrition, exercise, rest, minimizing stress and so forth. What I found was that all countries differed quite a bit from the norms of both the United States, and European ways of living.

The skin, our second largest organ of our body (fascia being the first despite the fact it is often ignored as an organ) is genetically endowed to withstand the climates and atmosphere of that part of the world from which they've historically originated or over time, adapted to.

Of course, over the centuries people have moved around from place to place, intermarried with people of other races, and sometimes moved to a geographical region different from that which their skins had genetically adapted in terms of safeguarding them from the elements typically found in a certain region.

These factors mean that "skin type for a specific region programmed for safeguarding by genetics" has essentially been undermined. In other words, the person now faces a skin type best suited for one region of world, while living in a region that requires something else entirely. That person's skin once had a genetic advantage for that region, but no longer. Genetic imprinting takes eons, meaning that those persons will have to adapt in other ways, such as use skin lotions, sun screens, protective hats and clothing and so on, to protect themselves from everything from not getting adequate exposure, to the sun to severe sunburns, to rare skin conditions including a variety of skin cancers.

That said, "base root of race" still exists, and the various chemical, histological and anatomical differences for all these changes, and especially as it relates to the care of the skin, medical procedures, and even the various ingredients within lotions, must be considered when addressing Asian skins, African skins, Caucasoid skins, and Indian skins (which in the southern parts of India are more sensitive and fragile despite the very deep tones). Is it any wonder that Mainland China has hundreds of billboards touting various skin whiteners.

I'm not in favor of skin whiteners, and thankfully, more and more we are accepting that the tone of our skin at birth is beautiful and should be the one with which we face the world. My view is that all skins should be their own natural and beautiful tone. As for the whiteners, I have heard and seen many horror stories of people trying to "bleach" their skin, using all kinds of acid peels and using too high percentages of hydroquinone and even laundry bleach packs. All this is dangerous and can cause varying degrees of trauma on the mechanisms responsible for triggering melanin in the first place.

As I said, the industry has been successfully treating hyperpigmentation in all its forms for decades, even sometimes getting results that seem magical. But it takes time. Most of all, it takes fundamental understanding of just how pigmentation works, where it comes from, and why we all have it in the first place!

Australia enjoys an increasingly growing Asian and Oriental community. People from Singapore, Malaysia and Hong Kong are increasingly migrating to Australia for vacations or to enjoy the Australian sun. Some own holiday homes there and visit as often as they can. Here's the thing: Oriental and Asian skins, by virtue of the yellow / brown pigmentation cells copiously endowed by nature, normally respond very well to sunlight. But the countries from where many of these people migrated are also humid with consistent precipitation in the air. In Australia, most areas are arid with very direct sunlight. The result is mass hyperpigmentation, dehydrated skins, dark spots, and accelerated wrinkles at just thirty-five years of age that you wouldn't normally expect to see until age sixty or so.

MELANIN CELLS

Contrary to the popular belief that Orientals and Asians possess more melanin cells than Caucasians (and black skins even more), everybody, regardless of race, possesses the same amount of melanin cells; they are just packaged differently.

The melanocyte (parent melanin cell) produces excess melanin whenever there is any trauma to the skin. This is true be it a passive trauma—such as chloasma (pregnancy mask)—or other hormonal changes or inflammatory hyperpigmentation such as caused by excessive sun damage, injury from outside the skin sources, or squeezing pimples and blemishes.

Oddly enough, the passive type hyperpigmentation is the most difficult to lessen, or remove.

Packaging of Melanin

Imagine the melanocytes as large egg-shaped cells surrounded by a large irregular triangle. The cell itself would occupy the bottom of the triangle and disperse pigment bearing melanin to little kidney-shaped cells near the top of the triangle. These kidney shaped receptacles are the actual melanin cells—and every race possess the same amount.

However, the pigmented material provided by the melanocyte and contained within each melanin cell, is very different from one race of people to another.

> Nature is smart and provides a reason and a way for the human body to work together for the well-being of the person.

Caucasian skin may have three little dots of pigment material inside the melanin cell. A black skin may have the entire cell filled with pigment material, while an Asian or Oriental skin will have three large dots of pigmented material within the melanin cell. This material has an ability to draw natural carotenes from the body into the cell as well, hence the yellowish color. Skin tone for Asians with vitamin A deficiencies, for example, can appear very pasty and dull in appearance.

Nature is smart and provides a reason and a way for the human body to work together for the well-being of the person. At the first sign of trauma, the melanocyte pumps pigment to the melanin cell as a line of skin defense against the trauma that is now attacking the young, basal layer cells of the skin. It will keep pumping pigment until it is exhausted, leaving an excess of pigmentation at the skin's surface that remains there indefinitely. The epidermis also becomes thickened in the trauma phase, building excess cuticle as an outward defense system, rather like a coat of armor.

The result is a pigmented hypertrophic scar with varying degrees of thickness.

TREATING HYPERPIGMENTATION

There are as many different treatments and claims of treatment for pigmentation disorders, as there are stars in the sky! Most treatments are based on bleaching away the redundant melanin using over-the-counter bleaching creams or quack treatments such as drinking copious amounts of lime water and Epsom salts.

Bleaching cream normally contains the drug Hydroquinone, which is an alkaloid of cinchona found in quinine sulfate mother liquors. Hydroquinone in 2% or less strength (the amount allowed by the Federal Drug Administration for use in cosmetics) is not particularly harmful when used sparingly, but it only temporarily suppresses pigmentation, which then comes back with a vengeance when that person goes out in the sun!

Stronger percentages of Hydroquinone, however, can become quite damaging and create severe pigmentation problems. In the Danné Montague-King Research Foundation in Singapore and South Africa, we've seen dreadful cases of ochronosis (very black, raised, almost burnt-looking hyperpigmentation), and skin cancers, due to over use of high percent Hydroquinone products.

Of course, prevention is the best policy, and a good transdermal grease-free sunblock that doesn't reek of coconut oil is the first thing you need. As for removal, that take weeks, even months. Everyone wants visible results right off the bat, of course. You would assume the pigmentation will disappear immediately, but this isn't the case. I can't tell you how many clients are very disgruntled when after the third week the spots are still there! This is because skin responds to new cell development in stages. Deep-seated pigmentation, especially the passive type that took years to develop, may take a little more time to fade or disappear completely.

Undoing the Damage

Rather than "spot treat" the dark area, my experience has been that every cell of the skin is interconnected. The first step would be to hydrolyze away the entire face, neck, and decollate area with at least three treatments using enzymes, alternated with low-level alpha hydroxy acid serums—the types that DO NOT depend on the unpredictable Glycolic acid for exfoliation. Oriental and Asian skins are particularly susceptible to any product containing Glycolic acid, so caution is warranted.

Once the dead and dying cuticle is removed, the pathway to the excess melanin is cleared. Many times, a great deal of this old melanin goes away in this initial hydrolyzing process. At DMK International, we use a unique system called the MELANOTECH SYSTEM that does not involve Hydroquinone.

You cannot naturally and safely lighten a person's skin beyond its normal pigmentation potential.

Many years ago I ran across a Japanese astringent / antiseptic ingredient from a botanical source, called *Kojic Acid*. I discovered that blending Kojic Acid with two other botanical ingredients not only dissembled old melanin (breaking it up literally) but helped to re-direct and regulate the normal flow of melanin to the traumatized area. This resulted in normal skin tone. After thirty-odd years in the professional skin treatment area, what I like to call the skin revision business, I realized I had stumbled onto a breakthrough.

The application of this formula is contained in 15 possible treatments for every type of hyperpigmentation, rosacea, and dark acne scarring. The formula itself comes in three strengths and in three different bases for professional and home use. Essentially, after the entire skin is denuded of its dead cell material, the serums and transdermal creams in the Melanotech Systems are applied to the dark pigment areas only.

This is especially important in Asian skin, as their normal skin tones have a habit of lightening up to their palest genetical potential, making the slower to respond hyperpigmentation look even darker for a while (although it will always catch up eventually).

There is one thing most people do not realize: You cannot naturally and safely lighten a person's skin beyond its normal pigmentation potential.

Post Treatment

During the entire phase of treatment, and after maximum results are achieved, the client must protect the entire face, neck, decollate, as well as the backs of their hands, with a transdermal sunblock.

Keeping the pH of the skin very low is also vital. Oriental skins should have an acid mantle on their skin of around 4.8 to maintain the new, bright even tone. This is accomplished by cleansing with an acid-based cleanser made of natural surfactants, such as soap barks, oak barks, century plant extract, Ritha plant, and other saponins.

Transdermal creams, water soluble containing at least 3% vitamin C are essential in not only maintaining this acid mantel but providing the living cells with the right amount of proteins after the dead cuticle is removed, thus keeping them alive a little longer (remember: all skin cells are interconnected). This is good news, in that if the normal pigmented cells are at maximum health, they will influence the unhealthy hyperpigmented cells next to them.

6

Hyperpigmentation: Causes and Treatments

Caucasians suffer from hyperpigmentation too, but their melasmas and "age spots" stand out even more than they do for people with deeper-tone skin. Most of the inflammatory pigmentation suffered is about solar damage from the sun, and can result in everything from simple tanning to basal cell carcinomas and other cancers.

It is interesting that the Asian preoccupation with having porcelain white skin comes from the days of the Emperor's and other members of The Imperial Court, all the way down to wealthy merchants and their wives and children. This group of Asian society were often over-weight and their skin being very pale. Such was a considered a plus, a sign of wealth and privilege. Being obese was proof they were rich enough to have all the delicacies they could consume; their pale skin a testament that they didn't have to toil in the sun as did the farmers and field laborers, who with their sparse and simple mainly vegetable diets, were mostly lean and muscular.

Caucasians typically strive for tan, lean and muscular. Aside from the fact that being lean is preferable to obesity for health reasons alone, if put in the context of "status," it could be said that "tan, lean and muscular" gives the air of someone who can afford a gym membership and the luxury of time to work out and maybe even with a personal trainer. Being lean could be construed as affording a diet of fresh vegetable, fruits, grains and meats, and being tan a sign of time or holidays on the sunny beaches of Hawaii or on yachts in the Mediterranean.

In both cases, the damages are the same.

How Melanin is Produced

It all starts at the Golgi apparatus (a complex of vesicles and folded membranes within the cytoplasm of most eukaryotic cells, involved in secretion and intracellular transport) which supplies pigmented cells to the melanocyte. Also referred to as the Golgi complex, it's part of the cell's endomembrane system.

Its primary function includes sorting and processing proteins. Proteins are synthesized in the rough endoplasmic reticulum, then they travel to the Golgi body.

What is not known about the melanocyte far outweighs the knowledge we do have available. Basically, the melanocyte is responsible for skin color. Human skin comes in four colors: red, yellow, brown and blue—though there may be hundreds of variations in between, should something go awry, such as Vitiligo. Top model, Chantelle Brown-Young, born to parents of Jamaican heritage contracted vitiligo at the age of four.

Vitiligo

Vitiligo, sometimes referred to as leucoderma is a chronic autoimmune disorder that causes a loss of pigment on sections of the skin. This de-pigmentation is not uniform, but manifests in blotches and patches around the body, particularly the face and hands. It occurs when melanocytes—the bodily cells responsible for skin pigment, die or cease functioning. The condition is non-contagious, but there is no cure. Vitiligo affects roughly two per cent of the population. It is not specific to black people, and affects all ethnicities, but is simply more visible as a result of their darker pigment. But note how popular Chantelle is today—and it is precisely because, thankfully we are beginning to respect and appreciate the skin's tone—whatever the color.

The melanocyte produces melanin granules. These melanosomes contain the material melanin. This brown pigment is transferred from the melanocyte to the keratinocytes in the granular layer of the skin. Only when the melanocyte enters the keratinocytes does the skin have color.

All races of people have nearly the same amounts of melanocytes available in their skins. But the melanin in each melanocyte is of a different amount. Caucasians have less melanin in their melanocytes than black-skinned people or Asian or Hispanic people. The amount of melanin in keratinocytes determines the degree of color in the skin or hair.

In the skin, there is one melanocyte to 35 keratinocytes, this is called EMU (epidermal melanocyte unit). The most important thing to know about melanin and skin pigmentation is that normal skin color, without exposure to radiation or hormone interaction, is called consecutive skin color. Inducible pigmentation that occurs with ultraviolet radiation, hormonal flux, or inflammation is called facular pigmentation, or hyperpigmentation.

The chemistry of melanin is complex, but there are two basic types of melanin that we need to know about. The first is eumelanin, a brown to black pigment that is a polymer of high molecular weight, its chemical composition is unknown, making it very difficult to study. The second is phaeomelanin, the yellow pigment that occurs only in the hair, except for certain Asian races where small amounts are in the skin.

With all the new tanning devices flooding the market, we must possess a basic understanding of the melanin process to better deal with the problems that may arise from overexposure, especially in wintertime when people tend to rely more on either fake tans (harmless) or sunbeds (mostly harmful).

TANNING AND MELANOGENESIS

There is no safe way to tan outside of artificial tans or tanning at such a slow degree that one turns only a slight bisque color after weeks of low-level tanning sessions. The effect of ultraviolet light on the melanocyte is not yet fully understood. Many years ago. when tanning beds were first popular, I would caution my patients to lie on them for only 30 minutes three times a week (15 minutes for very fair skinned people). But even then, I was doing them a disservice in the name of tanning popularity.

The aging and cancer-causing effects of solar damage, regardless of its source, are well known today. They may not show up at first if the person has strong or ethnic generation factors, but eventually the real story will come out. Even ethnic melanin genetic protection born to the deeper toned people of the world is no longer good enough, because our ozone layer is rapidly depleting its protective barrier, and over large sections of the planet.

The main controlling step in the synthesis of melanin is the conversion of tyrosine to dopa by the enzyme tyrosinase. It is at this point that we can insert our topical inhibitors with special skin treatments that literally stop the production of melanin. Anything that gets between tyrosine and tyrosinase can stop pigmentation temporarily.

Melanin Inhibitors

There are several natural and botanical sources of melanin inhibitors that interrupt between tyrosine and tyrosinase, such as Kojic acid (from fungus), mulberry, and nettle plants. Arbutin is another strong inhibitor and when precisely blended with other plant extracts, literally converts inside the skin to another type of bleaching action, like hydroquinone but without the possible toxic side effects often associated with this bleaching chemical.

We will be seeing more and more of this "conversion theory" where topically applied ingredients are transformed into another type of ingredient inside the skin. Enzymes already present in our skin physiology bring about this action/reaction.

Inhibiting pigmentation before it starts is not safely possible. I have had hundreds of people with beautiful, even-toned skin ask me if they could use pigmentation-inhibiting products whilst on holiday to avoid sun damage. I have always said no, keeping in mind that melanin being rushed to the epidermis during a state of trauma is a natural defense mechanism. Without this defense, radiation from the sun could kick-off cancer-causing effects in the skin, or trigger mass hyperpigmentation, as no one can cover the entire bodies with such as product at all time.

Inhibitors are great when treating hyperpigmentation, after you diagnose the type of pigmentation problems. Normally, hyperpigmentation is in isolated spots, or scattered over the face. Inhibitors should be applied to these areas only with special processes that could involve the use of ice or liquid nitrogen.

Freezing the area of pigmentation creates an "osmotic sink," which keeps the inhibition formulas trapped in the pigment area and does not influence the naturally colored skin around the spot. This will slow down or halt the formation of new melanin at that site whilst the old, dark pigmentation can be removed from the epidermis with enzyme treatments or other modalities that use either low or high pH products to quickly exfoliate the dead surface cells.

Treating Hyperpigmentation Safely

These types of treatments must be handled with speed and skill. Ironically, a lot of things that remove the problem of hyperpigmentation can also cause the problem if not performed correctly. It is essential to note that anything on the acid end of the pH scale used to remove dead cells and old, dark melanin must be 3.6 or under to work at all.

The better method, in my opinion, would be to alkalize the tissue with compounds that raise the pH of the skin to 12 on the pH scale. This totally desquamates all dead cells, and old melanin, in about four minutes.

Of course, this type of treatment is advanced. And, while effective in the hands of a trained therapist, it can also be dangerous. Over the years in the skin-care and skin-revision business, I have seen incredible results using alkaline—and almost equal amounts of horror stories.

Those suffering from hyperpigmentation usually view it as disfiguring—and many times it is. Pigmentation removal can take a long time if it is hormonal or drug induced from within the body. Inflammatory cases, however, disappear rapidly if handled correctly.

7

Scar Tissue, Revision and Treatments

Back in the 1960s when I started in the skin health industry, I never dreamed that deep and livid scars could be removed without surgery. In fact, even the best surgery is merely exchanging a bad scar with a lessor appearing scar. But I have had the honor of seeing really life altering scars totally removed without surgery! The good news is that quite a lot CAN be done as compared to the pampering, cleansing facials of yesteryear.

Take a look at our website, and you'll see some dramatic (and real) "before" and "after results: www.DMKCosmetics.com.

MEDICAL TREATMENT FOR SCARS

The way a scar develops depends as much on how your body heals, as it does on the original injury or the surgeon's skill. The variables that affect the severity of scarring include:
1. The size and depth of the wound;
2. The blood supply to the area;
3. The thickness and color of the skin (including ethnic aspects); and,
4. The direction of the scar on the skin (across or with the grain of the skin).

KELOID SCARS: Keloids are thick, puckered, itchy clusters of scars that grow beyond the edges of the wound or incision. They are often red or darker than the surrounding skin. Keloids appear when the body continues to produce collagen long after the initial wound healing has taken place. Keloids can appear anywhere on the body but are more common over the breastbone, earlobes and shoulders. Generally, Keloid scars lessens with age.

Treatment: Injections of steroid material directly into the scar tissue reduces redness, itching and sometimes shrinks the scar. Also, scar tissue can be cut out and the wound closed with one or two layers of stitches. Skin grafts are occasionally used if another Keloid develops after the revision surgery, but the donor site for the graft risks Keloids, as well.

No matter what approach is taken, Keloids have a stubborn tendency to recur, sometimes even larger than before. In these cases, the surgeon may combine the scar removal with direct steroid application during surgery or radiation therapy. Pressure garments are commonly prescribed by a physician in severe, recurring Keloids, and are worn for up to a year.

HYPERTROPHIC SCARS: These scars are often confused with Keloids since both appear to be thick, red or dark brown and raised. The difference is that hypertrophic scars remain within the boundaries of the original incision or wound. They often improve on their own in a year or two.

Treatment: Surgical removal of the excess scar tissue will involve repositioning the scar so that it reveals in a less visible manner. Steroid injections at the time of surgery, and at intervals for up to two years, help to prevent the thick scar from forming again.

BURNS / CONTRACTURES: Burns or injuries resulting in the loss of a large area of skin may form a scar that pulls the edges of the skin together, a process called contraction. This contraction could affect the muscles and tendons restricting normal movement.

Treatments: Correcting a contracture usually involves cutting out the scar and replacing it with a skin graft or flap. Z-Plasty may be used in some cases. **Z-Plasty** is a surgical technique used to reposition a scar so that it more closely conforms to natural lines and creases of the skin where it will be less noticeable. This procedure also frees up the tension on the skin and relieves the lack of movement in the area.

In Z-Plasty, the old scar is removed, and new incisions are made on each side, creating small triangular flaps of skin. These flaps are then rearranged to cover the wound at a different angle, giving the scar a Z pattern. The wound is then closed with very fine stitches.

In **Flap Surgery**, skin along with underlying fat, blood vessels and sometimes muscle, is moved from a healthy part of the body to the injured site. In some flap surgery the blood supply remains attached to one end of the donor site. In others, the blood vessels in the flap are reattached to the new site using micro vascular surgery.

In the case of highly visible facial scars, most that are not hypertrophic can simply be cut out after the initial wound is healed and re-stitched with fine stitches resulting in a finer, smaller scar that fades with time. If the scar lies along natural creases or lines in the face, Z plasty is often employed in the scar revision surgery.

Many physicians follow up these revision techniques with dermabrasion to smooth the skin, especially in the case of keloids or hypertrophic scars, but I have never seen a case where dermabrasion completely removed a scar.

NON-MEDICAL TREATMENTS FOR SCARS

Scar tissue is still skin tissue. It has become scar tissue because the injury has caused the desmosomes to release new cells to surface much faster than the patient's natural new cell proliferation (so much for cosmetic products claiming to accelerate new skin cells!).

Scar tissue, like normal skin can, be softened, partially removed and de-pigmented. Keep in mind, however, that the following techniques take time, very much like the time it takes a jeweler to tap away at a rough diamond to bring out a clean facet.

Microdermabrasion: Continuous treatments using a microdermabrader results in a planning down of hypertrophic scar tissue. However, this should be considered ONLY as a tool for opening the door to further treatment.

Light Treatment: There are claims that certain wavelengths of light can not only remove signs of aging, but can also remove scars. Laser skin revision (laser also being a form of light) can assist in scar revision, but these treatments require the use of a MEDICAL laser.

Electromagnetic Energy Treatments: The incredible re-polarizing powers of pulsing electromagnetic waves can be programmed like a computer for very quick post-surgical wound healing. This type of treatment can be performed immediately after the physician has completed a scar revision procedure. Better yet, electromagnetic waves appear to regulate normal cell proliferation, which is vital to keloid revision. I have seen unbelievable examples of success using this approach on the tissues of the body.

Alkalizing the Tissues: There are water-soluble compounds available that raise the pH of the skin to around 12 on the pH scale. Alkalizing the skin correctly softens and dissolves the scar tissue creating a mild irritation that forms a light scab. When the scab falls off, the scar appears flatter. Extreme care must be used to avoid excessive trauma that might lead to additional scaring and/or pigmentation problems.

Enzyme Skin Tightening Treatments: Scars on aging skin tend to look deeper or more predominant as the skin loosens with age, particularly in the case of ice pick acne scars. Tightening the skin with enzyme treatments gives a temporary but progressive lift to the tissues, which also smooths out the appearance of scars as the skin becomes firmer. This would be like smoothing out wrinkles on a bed spread by pulling the corners tight.

Acidic Oils: There are some oils on the market from both the marine world and the botanical world that soften and flatten scars and reduce dark pigmentation. No one is really one hundred percent sure why these types of oils work (I have my theories of course) but many wonderful results have been observed over the years. The oil I am most familiar with is from the **Rosa Mesquita Oil** from Chile and many of its cousins. These oils must be applied at least three times a day directly on the scar tissue and they must be fractionated enough to enter the tissues.

Most of the work I have personally been involved with the past few decades regarding scar revision has involved all the above methods, often used in various combinations on each client. The main thing with scar revision treatments is PATIENCE. Skin CAN be molded like living plastic; it can be made to respond with chemistry, electromagnetic therapy, and surgery. But successful scar revision takes time.

Skin CAN be molded like living plastic; it can be made to respond with chemistry, electromagnetic therapy, and surgery.

8

The "Dry Martini" Approach to Advertising Skin Health Products

I started venturing into the holistic field in the 1960's. Even then I thought of it as "WHOLISTIC" (meaning the whole body, and from the inside, out), conscious of the fact that good health relies a good deal on healthful personal habits, such as nutrition, exercise and sleep.

Personally, I was doing the Atkins Low Carb diet years before Dr. Atkins became a household name. There was a little sandwich shop behind my very first clinic near the beach, and I would order sandwiches with sprouts, tuna, beef, chicken or turkey, and mayonnaise, but no bread! Bread of almost any kind—except sourdough which has an enzyme that very slowly releases carbohydrates into your body—always made me feel puffy and bloated, especially in the stomach area, creating a "muffin top" at my waistline when wearing snug jeans. As a result, I would ask for hard slabs of Swiss Cheese in substitution for bread.

This always worked and I have stayed on a low carb diet for most of my life. What is in the gut can show up in the skin, and in many cases, is the root cause of skin disorders, aside from acne which is mostly hormonal (although a bad diet can influence insulin and exacerbate acne).

INSIDE OUT: Wholistic Vs. Holistic Living

Ever wonder how a vitamin company manages to cram a dozen different ingredients into one tiny pill? The truthful answer is, they can't! This is what I call the "dry martini" approach. The company takes the latest sexy sounding ingredient (like Alpha Lipoic Acid or DHEA) and puts a miniscule amount of it in the formula, for the sole purpose of advertising it on the label. Then they create hype around the ingredient on advertising campaigns even though clinical studies show you need ten times the level indicated to get any health benefits.

There is also a lot of corner-cutting, such as using less-expensive herbal powders instead of the more effective extracts or herbs that have not been standardized. Binders and fillers are added in such amounts that effect the way the product dissolves into your body and is absorbed.

The good news is that there are a lot of supplements out there that are highly effective in getting better results from your topical skin treatments. Even better news is that therapists who can run highly detailed panels from saliva, fecal material and urine, can let you know what is going on INSIDE that results in skin problems we view on the outside.

The brain ultimately controls everything and sends signals to the hypothalamus gland to relay messages of stress or energy that can affect the entire hormonal cascade in men and women which then ends up in the skin. There are very few "brain food" products that rejuvenate brain cells and fire up the synapses. Taken properly, the few that really work as seemingly miracle ingredients can also speed up memory and learning retention, reverse mental dullness, brain fog and, cognitive decline.

All of these have been subjected to numerous case studies and have few, if any, side effects if taken in the right dosages. The first one is phosphatidyl serine, a naturally occurring fat found in young, healthy brains.

Alpha-Glyceryl Phosphorylcholione:
A Building Block for the Brain

Alpha-Glyceryl Phosphorylcholione (ALPHA-GPC) is a special form of choline that is a building block in the brain that helps produce chemical messengers called "neurotransmitters" that boost cognitive performance. The "alarm clock" for your brain (wakes it up for better thinking and longer attention span) is Acetyl-L-Carnitine. Vinpocetine is a vasodilator that relaxes the capillaries of the brain and enhances circulation. Like Acetyl-L-Carnitine, it is a powerful antioxidant that can repair free radical damage IN the brain immediately.

The last best-brain-food outside of the common need for essential fatty acids found in fish are Evening Primrose Oil, Seabuckthorn Oil, and common Blueberries. Not only do blueberries taste great, but they have the highest levels of free radical fighters compared to over forty fruits and vegetables.

The antioxidant powers of blueberries are twenty times greater than tomatoes and ten times greater than beta-carotene. Blueberries are also packed with anthocyanins, a potent flavonoid that contains four times the free radical scavenging abilities of vitamin C.

Cortisol

Among the many things instigated by hormonal flux that can contribute to acne, rosacea, eczema, dermatitis and premature aging skin, are Cortisol levels. Cortisol controls many things in the skin and body.

Cortisol is a cortisteroid hormone produced by the adrenal gland. It has often been referred to as "the stress hormone." Keeping cortisol levels balanced is necessary for successful skin revision treatments for those who are chronically inflamed or broken out. Out of balance cortisol levels can create high blood pressure and lower the immune response. It can also inhibit collagen production in the skin and weaken muscles.

Cortisol and the Electromagnetic Wave Machine

Balanced cortisol levels can reduce stress (so necessary during acne treatments), restore homeostasis, and stimulate superoxide dismutase for maximum skin immunity. It is also acts as a "poison" against bacterial infection.

The only sure-fire way I know to regulate cortical during skin revision treatments, is the use of pulsing electromagnetic wave machines. Precisely programmed, this type of apparatus can deliver the exact amount of pulses per minute at the right frequencies, intensities and so on. And, it will immediately repolarize traumatized cells in the body and skin, reinstate our natural electromagnetic fields, and, stimulate the hypothalamus gland into correcting out-of-control cortisol levels.

Electromagnetic wave therapy does a great deal more than that, but I have seen incredible and quick results with inflamed skin conditions on very hard cases when EMW machines were used in tandem with a good, topical treatment. One of the best is put out by CURATIVE, an Australian based company. Entitled the DERMAFIELD, this machine is used widely by plastic surgeons and dermatologists pre- and post-surgery for maximum and rapid healing and no scars. It has recently become available for beauty therapists who specialize in age management, acne and problematic skin conditions.

Bad Brain Food vs Good Brain Food

There has been a lot of hype on the following ingredients or products to the point that serious researchers have performed exhaustive tests to show how dangerous these ingredients really can be—amongst them are Phenytoin, Fipexide, and the poorly monitored HGH (Human Growth Hormone).

Phenytoin (Dilantin) is commonly used for epilepsy victims. This anticonvulsant is falsely promoted as a "brain and IQ booster." It is not, and in fact has serious side-effect potentials, everything from slurred speech and insomnia, to deadly liver disorders, blood defects and dodgy thyroids.

Fipexide. The over-the-counter stimulant is supposed to enhance thinking and learning by increasing the dopamine levels of the brain, making us "think younger thus act younger." There is some evidence in one trial, that mental functioning was slightly improved in a group of patients with brain disease. But, it also can cause severe liver damage.

Stay away from this one!

Human Growth Hormone (HGH). I wish this protein secreted by the pituitary gland that promotes cell growth did NOT grow potential tumors or other cancer cells in the body, but it can have that effect. Many people may have cancer potential cells in their bodies that remain benign and never develop for nearly a lifetime. HGH will develop them, and as rapidly as it develops young cells in the body!

HGH is still too iffy to recommend to anyone. There is a lot of "fake" HGH out there—so-called "natural" over-the-counter supplements and even some very suspect medically injected offerings.

All of them are a waste of money.

I have experimented with injectable HGH and a proven oral spray. The results were negligible and not worth the high cost. I feel that the Live Cell Therapy I have been having once a year since 1984 gives a far better result of well-being, energy and more youthful body tissue.

DHEA. This steroid hormone produced by the adrenal gland is touted as an "anti-aging" nutrient that helps you age more gracefully. It really does work (internally, not in a beauty crème), but without a Doctor's supervision the risks may outweigh the benefits. Women taking DHEA are prone to "masculine" side-effects like unnatural hair growth and a deepening voice and weight gain. Men can develop "man boobs" or breast tenderness. There is the possibility of frightening side effects such as heart palpitations, altered blood sugar levels and increased cancer risk. In short do not take DHEA unless under a doctor's supervision.

Gerovital. Discovered by Ana Aslan in Romania decades ago, Gerovital has been sold to millions as the ultimate anti-aging supplement. Before FDA approval as a supplement (only deemed as safe to take, not categorized as effective in which case it would have to be a drug), I used to see tons of this product smuggled into the USA by multi-level schemes or quack anti-aging doctors and "health specialists." There is no scientific evidence whatsoever that Gerovital rejuvenates anything at all. It really is nothing more than the local anesthetic procaine, combined with an antioxidant and a preservative.

DRUGS AND SKIN

The skin's pH and even cell structure can be altered by prescription drugs. This is important to know before undergoing any resurfacing peels or deeper microdermabrasion. Likewise, the aesthetic doctor or clinician should be aware of these before performing any laser resurfacing, photo facials and the new over hyped, Fraxel treatments.

The most important one to look out for is RO-Accutane.

Accutane being a vitamin A derivative, has side effects that are like Hypervitaminosis, a toxic syndrome from excess intake of vitamin A. First, Accutane inhibits the production of sebum in the skin. This is dose related, which means the more medication you take and the longer you take it, the more reduction of sebum. Eventually your skin will not produce sebum, so that the skin will become cracked and dry and need external support.

A common side effect is chronic dry lips and thin, red skin subject to hyper pigmentation when exposed the even minimal sunlight. But these symptoms are not as severe as the fact that extended use of Accutane decreases the enzyme collagenase in the skin, which is essential to the proper reconstruction of skin when it is irritated, traumatized, cut into—or resurfaced in any way that is more than the mildest facial.

When the collagen enzyme is not functioning normally, scaring can occur at any time when the skin is broken and needs to heal. Scaring has been reported in 49% of the patients taking Accutane and can last up to seven years after Accutane treatments have been stopped. The labs that produce the drug also warn of Pseudotumor Cerbri (benign increase of pressure on the brain) as another side effect. The list goes on.

Coumadin

Coumadin, a blood thinner drug is also dangerous in that it prevents clotting but increases the danger of bleeding, bruising and interferes with vitamin K, essential to healthy capillaries—the very conduits of nutrients we need carried to the mitochondria in our skin cells.

These are but a few of the drugs to be aware of.

On the flip side, there is a list of supplements KNOWN to benefit skin health. I call this my "BASIC WELLNESS LIST" and it is a regimen I take myself. It is by no means conclusive for everyone and as always, check with your physician or a medically qualified person to be sure they are right for you. Again, the partial list below is compiled for the IU (potency needed) of each ingredient the body requires for maximum internal health.

Suppliements Know to Benefit Skin Health

Vitamin A	15,000 IU
Vitamin C	10,000 IU
Magnesium	400 IU
Vitamin D	300 IU
Vitamin E	500 IU
Vitamin B1	75 mg
Vitamin B2	50 mg
Vitamin B3	150 mg
Vitamin B6	102 mg
Folic Acid	800 MCG
Vitamin B12	250 mcg
Biotin	400 mcg
Pantothenic Acid	500 mg

Calcium	282 mg
Iodine	10 mcg
Zinc	20 mg
Manganese	25 mg
Chromium	200 mg
Selenium	200 mcg
Molybdenum	125 mcg
Potassium	50 mg
Copper	2 mg
Evening Primrose Oil	515 mg
Seabuckthorn Oil	515 mg

Keep in mind that dosage is important, as well as knowing the best time of day to ingest it. Should it be taken with or without meals, and so on. There is only ONE all-in-one product, that I am aware of, that is easier to take and that is REGENERADE, developed by world famous cell therapy scientist Sir Thomas Smith, MD.

Dr. Smith's formulation is patented and has a unique enzymatic delivery system that promotes total delivery and absorption into the body and skin cells, however this product is available through health professionals only and dosages vary depending on your age and physical condition. Again, check with a pharmacist or health professional.

9

The Glycation Rage: Why Sugar Makes Us Look Older

In the late 1980s the big rage in aging skin was to blame sugar, which resulted in the term GLYCOSYLATION. Oddly enough, the cosmetic industry did not jump on this one with a plethora of miracle products like the wellness gurus did with their war on consuming sugar. My mother was diabetic and was in all kinds of University research programs up in Seattle, Washington. They were using all kinds of new ingredients to either neutralize excess glucose in diabetics or convert it into harmless energy.

One of those ingredients interested me, so I burned a lot of midnight oil trying to figure out which of its variations would also negate the excess glucose in skin that cause crossed-linked wrinkles!

Only one form of this ingredient would work. The other two forms could be highly reactive and volatile. It really was a roll of the dice and a toss of the coin. Or an educated guess. In any case, we stopped glycosylation in its tracks!

My early research can begin with an idea totally unrelated to another idea, yet both ideas end up on common ground! So how does the research regarding how to deter collagen deficiency in the aorta of laboratory rats, and how to offset some of the extreme symptoms of adult on-set diabetes, end up in a therapy on prohibiting cross-linked wrinkles on human skin?

Fortunately, like-minded scientific seekers sometimes get together and compare notes here in the USA, and as a result, quite often thus a new treatment is born! The phenomenon I am referring to is, "glycosylation."

The Maillard Reaction

Meat browns, thus we brown because of glucose, the other major molecule of aerobic metabolism. This peculiar phenomenon was discovered in 1912 by Louis Maillard, a French chemist, who observed that a mixture of glucose to protein components, when heated, would turn from clear to yellow to a deep brown. This was subsequently called the *Maillard Reaction* and has ever since been of great interest to food chemists concerned with making food as tasty and tempting in appearance as possible. The Maillard Reaction is just the chemical attachment of glucose to proteins at places it doesn't normally belong, which makes a yellow brown product. Glucose is sticky stuff, so it attaches spontaneously, given the appropriate temperature and amount of time.

Until recently, however, no one understood that this same process could occur at any body temperature. But in the 1970s it was noticed that people who have high levels of blood glucose due to poorly controlled diabetes, also have glucose attached to some of their hemoglobin, a protein. That is, their hemoglobin is modified as if by a Maillard Reaction. Doctors had noticed for years that uncontrolled diabetics seemed to undergo something resembling accelerated aging.

Advanced Glycosylation End-Products

Many of the common ailments of aging, such as cataracts, atherosclerosis, heart attacks, strokes, lung problems, and joint stiffening, appeared earlier in diabetics together with the Maillard Reaction. It was concluded that aging itself might be partially due to Maillard, or browning, or products accumulating at a slow rate in the body. What's more, Louis Maillard noted that the result of this reaction was a series of unalterable new chemical structures in our tissues, which he called AGEs, a clever acronym from his opaque chemical term, Advanced Glycosylation End-products.

But why would simply attaching glucose to proteins at places it doesn't belong, lead to the sort of deterioration we call aging? The first reason is that some proteins form the structure and support of our bodies. Many of the most important structural proteins, such as collagen, live for decades in our bodies without their molecules turning over. Apparently general characteristics of aging take place in exactly those tissues that are stuffed with long-lived, non-renewing cells and molecules.

Let's think about collagen again. Remember that it is a flexible protein composed of three strands coiled around one another like a cable. Its flexibility is what makes it so useful for forming the foundation of arteries, veins, lungs, and skin for making tendons and ligaments that twist and bend without breaking—and, for forming cartilage that cushions our joints with its resiliency. But as glucose attaches to collagen, it forms bridges or cross-links between strands of a single molecule and between molecules.

As these bridges multiply over time, collagen's flexibility gradually disappears. It turns yellow and stiff and no longer makes such wonderful lungs, tendons, ligaments, or support for artery walls. What's more, collagen with attached glucose in the walls of the arteries acts like an opened-jawed bear trap: it seizes and holds onto passing proteins. In this fashion, browning may play a part in trapping and accumulation of LDL cholesterol in the artery walls—an early stage of atherosclerosis.

The All-Important Proteins

Proteins do many things in the body besides provide its body structure. They turn genes on and off, direct cell replication, and chaperone other molecules to their appropriate site of action. As enzymes, they are essential for virtually all the chemical activity of a cell. The fidelity with which proteins carry out the functions they were designed for, depends on their being chemically unaltered. When sugars attach to protein inappropriately, they can impair their function and therefore disrupt the proper working of the cell. Attached sugars also make proteins less soluble in the body and more likely to solidify and become non-functional, and less likely to be broken down by chemicals designed to destroy damaged molecules.

The impairment of proteins isn't the only potential problem associated with glucose. Glucose can also bind directly to DNA, although it does so more slowly than it binds to proteins. Nevertheless, in non-dividing cells, such as those which compose much of the brain and heart, DNA is a long-lived molecule on which AGEs can potentially accumulate. In principle, AGE Attachment to DNA could disrupt the production of new cellular proteins, could interfere with DNA repair, and could even cause mutations. As of now, however, not enough is known about these processes.

Chemical theorists tell us that the Maillard Reaction should proceed at a rate pretty much determined by the concentration of sugars and proteins, and the temperature at which these ingredients are kept. To simplify, the same browning reactions that occurs when you cook meat on high heat takes place at a much slower rate on long-lived proteins in our bodies, principally collagen (the Maillard reaction). This initiates a glucose-driven intrinsic aging process.

Once this excess sugar enters the circulation it attaches itself to the amino groups of protein tissues such as collagen and rearranges the youthful structures into damaging demons called advanced glycation end products, or AGEs. These hardened molecules, sticky with excess glucose, cross link with other fibers such as elastin and cross-link, forming hard bridges that lead to prolapsed tissue and deep furrow or lines in the skin.

Newer studies showed that glycation of collagen increases with age. Fibroblast cell activity slows down, and a new phenomenon appears. A specific receptor called RAGE pulls the glycation process into the remaining fibroblast cells that are the literal factories of new collagen, compromising the tissue even further. In addition, glycation increases the release of collagen destructive enzymes known as MMP-1 and skin regeneration slows to a crawl.

We know that certain natural plant compounds, as well as synthetic drugs, can inhibit the formation of browning products in a test tube. So, it seems likely that our bodies will also contain an array of anti-browning chemicals, although they are yet unknown. But at least one of the body's phagocytes, or scavenger cells, seems specialized to devour proteins or cells that have been "browned."

If oxidation and browning are two important genera in processes of aging, it might come as no surprise that they seem to operate cooperatively to our detriment. The damage caused by one affects the other. So, glucose and its derivative products can react with other chemicals to produce free radicals, and free radical can accelerate browning. Also, glucose can attach to cellular antioxidant enzymes and by doing so inactivate them leading to higher levels of free radicals and the damage they cause.

Glycosyl: The Free Radical Not Recognized by the Cell

This is the original term we used years ago when we started research on AGEs. It starts with carbohydrates that we get from plants and animals when we eat. All carbohydrates are eventually broken down in the body into simple sugars or glucose, which can then take part in our energy producing metabolic processes. However, excess carbohydrates not immediately needed by the body are stored in the liver and the muscles of the body in the form of glycogen. If the glycogen is not used it becomes stagnant, rather like a pool of water that has no current running through it (a swamp) and at this point glycogen becomes a glycoside which produces glycosyl.

Glycosyl is a free radical that is not recognized as a nutrient by living cells, including skin cells. In addition to this damage by this evil free radical, another process takes place. Stagnant glycol, like stagnant water, begins to grow microorganisms. These are in the form of sticky little barnacles that glue the protein bonds that form healthy skin cells together so they cannot proliferate naturally. Malfunctioning cell proliferation leads to the collapse of collagen fibers and elastin, and this means sagging skin!

Along with the sag comes a whole plethora of malfunctions due to the advance of another free radical added to the invasive army of common free radicals. These vampires of healthy cell electrons take the attention of the skin's defense system away from having to help maintain a healthy skin. Now they must put all their energies into keeping the skin from breaking down completely! The result: DEEP CROSS-LINKED WRINKLES! Often seen on clients prematurely in their forties, these wrinkles resemble congealed gravy left in the fridge for a week! They can be also viewed on the back of the neck and hands or draped Austrian style around the neck.

The free radicals of sun damage do play a role in this as well, creating the free radical soup, lipofuscin, but Glycosylation surrounding the skin cells like a miasmic marsh loaded with eroding little microorganisms, is the new villain on the scene.

In addition to all the other dead cell removal systems my company has researched over the years, and the hydration and nutrient protein products that clients can put into their skins as rebuilding tools plus the addition of absorbable ascorbic acids to help support the collagen fibers, there was not much else that was known about how to circumvent glycosylation.

Aminoguanidine

In the early part of 1996, at DMK International, we became aware of a little ingredient called aminoguanidine (hydrasinecarboximidamide) which was originally tested as a prevention of glucose-derived collagen cross-linkage of the aorta of diabetic rats. But what really grabbed my interest was the research being done on human diabetics—in as much as my own Mother had a terrible case of onset adult diabetes to the point her feet almost had to be amputated! She underwent aminoguanidine research therapy and her problem reversed dramatically as far as the necrosis of the tissue was concerned (aminoguanidine and its precursors are not claimed to be cures for diabetes).

I also discovered that out of the three forms of aminoguanidine available, one was excellent in helping to stop glycosylation in aging skin.

Over the years we have observed that formulating certain ingredients into a spray or "spritz" application maximized their efficiency 75%. A fine, water-based mist sprayed over the skin mocks the action of the skin's own glands, the sudoriferous or sweat glands. This forms a "mantle" which in turn, can be sealed in with fractionated natural oil, such as DMK's Seba E oil. A water-soluble crème would be the final step, thus allowing all the active ingredients in the mist a longer time in the skin, which decreases the possibility of early evaporation.

This has proven to be very effective in not only stopping or slowing down the cross-linked wrinkling process, but brings a fresh, pink bloom to the pallid, grey skins of heavy smokers.

There was a study in Norway in 1999 that was so positive that they were calling it "the gold water." The Norwegians reported that after two weeks usage of aminoguanidine spray, applied under vitamin C crèmes or OPC crèmes (antioxidant crèmes), results in a firming and toning of the skin process that accelerates with each day used.

Since then, DMK research shows that Blueberries eaten or compounded into trans epidermal products, along with pomegranate extracts, carnosine, pyridoxal5-phosphate and benefotiamine, also act as powerful "anti-glycation" barriers. However, once the glycation is stopped, the deep fissures and lines in the skin remain and other types of skin resurfacing treatments and tissue building must be done again.

Beware of machines or products that claim to banish glycation totally. This is a CHEMICAL matter that must be addressed internally, life style habits of sunbathing changed to abstinence, and the AGEs negated by the specific free radical fighters.

10

The Key Powerful Healing Vitamins

Vitamin A has already surfaced as a peeling agent, touted as being superior to Alpha Hydroxy Acids. However, Vitamin A and its sisters Retinal (the most powerful exfoliant), Retinol, Resorcin, Resorcinol, and Retinoic Acid have been around for over thirty years and have been presented medically and cosmetically in different forms over that time period—including the past-popular Retin A (Tretinoin).

Vitamin A

The action of any of the Vitamin A's versus Alpha Hydroxy Acid is totally different, although they both "peel." Vitamin A compounds, lotions and the like, will help rebuild skin tissue over a period, whilst AHAs basically only remove via hygroscopic action, which ultimately dehydrates the skin and leads to acid hardened skin and thinner tissue. There have been huge claims that AHAs "lay down new collagen" in the skin (whatever that means). But we have noted in our AHA research that the new collagen formation starts at the point of after care (after AHA exfoliation) when Vitamin C treatment enters the picture.

> Oxidation appears to be involved in all skin diseases including aging.

I have worked with outstanding formulas based on the Vitamin A family that have rivalled laser skin resurfacing and without any of the contra-indications associated with YAG or CO2 lasers. I have been advocating the necessity of Vitamin C as a precursor to collagen stimulation through the fibroblast cells for years, yet it seems to be consistently advertised as an antioxidant being its main feature. It must take second place to another vitamin in the antioxidant army, which is Vitamin E.

Oxidation, Free Radicals and Oxidative Stress

Oxidation appears to be involved in all skin diseases including aging. This also involves atoms which are grouped into molecules which are the components of living cells. All cells in the skin, indeed in the body, require oxygen, amino acids and proteins as nutrients. A by-product of cellular respiration is the formation of a species of oxygen called Free radicals (discovered by Denham Harman in 1981).

Free radicals are unstable atoms that can damage cells, causing illness and aging.

Free radicals are linked to aging and a host of diseases, but little is known about their role in human health, or how to prevent them from making people sick. Free radicals are thought to be responsible for age-related changes in appearance, such as wrinkles and gray hair.

Understanding free radicals requires a basic knowledge of chemistry.

It's helpful to understand that atoms are surrounded by electrons that orbit the atom in layers called shells. Each shell needs to be filled by a set number of electrons. When a shell is full, it begins filling the next shell. If an atom has an outer shell that is not full, it may bond with another atom, using the electrons to complete its outer shell. These types of atoms are known as free radicals.

Atoms with a full outer shell are stable, but free radicals are unstable and inn effort to make up the number of electrons in their outer shell, they react quickly with other substances. When oxygen molecules split into single atoms that have unpaired electrons they become unstable free radicals that seek other atoms or molecules to bond to. If this continues to happen, it begins a process called oxidative stress.

Oxidative stress can damage the body's cells, leading to a range of disease and causes symptoms of aging, wrinkles being a minor example.

These destructive atoms with un-paired electrons are on a kamikaze mission to steal an electron from a nearby molecule. This destructive process results in oxidation, the rusting of cells.

Antioxidants are the antidote to these free radicals. Antioxidants donate electrons and render the free radicals harmless. This is an important preventive measure in skin treatments, as Free radicals cause the DNA strands to break and the mitochondria (intercellular structures) to lose their energy source—which is Aden triphosphate (ATP).

When this happens, the cells involved die and aging progresses rapidly.

Vitamin E & C

The first line of defense in the antioxidant army as mentioned above would be the tocopherols or Vitamin E, not Vitamin C. Both Vitamin A and E are fat soluble vitamins.

Vitamin E is the primary antioxidant for lipid membranes in the skin, mainly fatty acid membranes that comprise the photo receptors. Water soluble Vitamin C is also important but acts more like a scavenger of free radicals that have broken through the lipid bones of Vitamin E.

Oddly enough, in proper skin treatment a therapist would apply Vitamin C serum products on the skin first—which in turn would be occluded and kept in place, without much evaporation, by lipid rich Vitamin E. However, the important amino acid Glutathione must also be included in the treatment somewhere—either in an enzyme-based mask or a crème as a free radical prevention agent. Glutathione donates electrons to Vitamin C, Vitamin C donates to Vitamin E, recycles back to Glutathione in a complete, protective circle. The free radicals haven't a chance!

In addition to being a primary collagen enhancer and a secondary antioxidant, Vitamin C has another special talent: it is vital in the treatment of hyperpigmented or uneven toned skin. I observed many years ago while on a trip to the Southern State of Georgia, women rubbing lemons on their faces; their claim was that this simple home cosmetic was bleaching their skin. Likewise, my own mother rubbed lemons on her elbows every night for the same reason.

Kojic Acid: In researching ingredients that slowed down or prohibited excess melanin in the skin, I discovered that lemon inhibits the formation of tyrosinase in the skin far better than Kojic Acid or licorice root extract, mulberry leaf extract and all the other skin lightening botanicals put together. Vitamin C really does help remove pigmentation problems if formulated and administered correctly.

Citric Acid: Another humble cousin to Vitamin C, but a different ingredient is Citric Acid. This plain, natural ingredient was mainly used as a preservative in foods and cosmetics, until we uncovered the fact that it helps to increase dermal hydration via the chondroitin which helps to smooth and plump up thin, ageing skin! I have always included citric in my AHA formulas to help maintain hydration during dramatic AHA in clinic treatments.

Beta Glucan: A third winning ingredients publicity, Beta Glucan, has enjoyed almost as much ingredient publicity, at least in the USA, as vitamins for the skin. Beta Glucan directly enhances the Immune System of the skin through the stimulation of the Langerhans Cells located in the epidermis. For many, these cells were almost unknown to the skin care and skin revision industry. Almost everyone was led to believe that all true cell activity and life forces started in the dermis. But the epidermis is the first line of defense for the entire body and has many active components of its own, including the ignored Langerhans cells.

One of the first research projects establishing the effects of Beta Glucan was performed in the 1950's. A report in the journal "Cancer" showed a single dose of Beta glucan in test animals revved up their immunity. Low doses of this substance can help macrophages (octopus-like blobs in tissue with tentacles that can grasp infectious invaders in a depth grip) overcome tumors and infections associated with skin cancer, acne, eczema, among others.

In our studies at DMK International designed to boost immune cell activity, we have found that beta 1, 3 and 6D-glucan (1, 3-D-Glucan extracted from the cell walls of baker's yeast) have been clinically shown to stimulate the Langerhans cells which in turn act as receptors to the macrophage immune cells. This is vital for post laser treatments when the client is as red as a fall sunset, or after a particularly nasty sunburn. Sunburns are insults to the skin that are permanently recorded even in youth—something that really catches up to us from age forty, onward.

However, beta glucan erases this memory, if applied to the skin at least one-half hour after the burn! We're just now understanding not only its protective qualities but how to get the raw material at a reasonable rate so that products containing beta glucan are available to everyone. The original suppliers heavily armed with USA patents, charged an arm and a leg, but I get my suppliers from the fishing industry in the Scandinavian countries.

MICRODERMABRASION

Nothing has hit the skin care industry and the medical industry like Microdermabrador machines. Yet (in my opinion) they are just another tool in the physician's or the advanced therapist's kit bag.

Unfortunately, much like the AHA hoopla of the early 90s, Microdermabrasion is being touted as a miracle skin resurfacing treatment all on its own. Some tabloids credit the Microdermabrador as being able to remove stretch marks, lift faces, peel skin painlessly (yeah, right), and remove all wrinkles during a lunch break. In fact, the USA abounds with "lunch break" medical procedures lately, including laser. One would wonder what kind of jobs people had that would enable them to reappear at 2.00 pm with red, swollen faces grimacing in pain. I prefer the old fashioned three martini lunch myself—at least the red face is gone by nightfall.

> The key to using products containing vitamins and machines that remove human tissue is to check out the source thoroughly.

The original Microdermabrador was invented in Italy by Mattioli Engineering Company, who also manufacture fine laser equipment for the medical field. Entitled the Harvey Crystal, this Microdermabrador addressed the main complaint doctors have had for years against the conventional diamond fraise or wire brush dermabrasion—the field of blood that veiled the surface of the skin making it difficult for the doctors to see where they were going!

The Harvest Crystal possessed a unique patented glass hand piece that had two functions. The top part of the hand piece (which looks rather like a trombone) shot out a stream of natural, antiseptic Corundum crystals at high speed—which abraded the surface of the skin. The abraded tissue (and blood) was then immediately sucked back into the bottom portion of the hand piece and back into a special receptacle.

The machine operated off an adjustable compressor

allowing the operator to have full control of how much tissue was removed at one sitting. This was a very effective (albeit not painless) procedure.

Eventually the company modified the Harvest Crystal for use by beauty therapists. I saw this demonstrated in Norway around that time and wondered if they could get it passed by the Federal Drug Administration in the USA. They did, and thousands of test dollars later and four year's waiting time, then had their FDA number ripped off by an unscrupulous distributor who was selling to doctors in the USA before he realized that bigger money was in the beauty therapy field, where therapists outnumber physicians.

This is a definite place for Microdermabrasion—if the equipment is good, well-engineered with a warranty and the person using it is trained. It is invaluable in the removal of stretch marks, it does open the door very quickly to advance treatments of wrinkles, acne scars and pigmentation—in tandem with other treatments that involve active, botanical chemistry, but beware of promises of incredible results overnight with no pain.

The real Microdermabrador are highly engineered with complex parts that's must be handled properly. Training is vital for maximum results and little organic crystals must be 100% Corundum, not aluminum powder or synthetic "cheaper" brands. These types of abrasives just don't do the job and can be contraindicative to the client.

The key to using products containing vitamins and machines that remove human tissue is to check out the source thoroughly. Good science always has a definite logic behind it; it is not esoteric or evasive in concept. The concept is the philosophy behind the product and the philosophy must make sense in the grand scheme of things.

After all, the knee-bone is connected to the thigh bone!

11

Cells Within Cells: Injectables, Fillers and Threads

For many years I have talked about the living skin cell by comparing it to a medieval walled city. In the center of the city is the King in his castle (DNA) his Queen (Transfer RNA) and a Princess (Messenger RNA). Around the castle are warehouses where amino acids and other proteins are stored to feed the Royal Family. Elsewhere is the power station that energizes the city, the all-important mitochondria and finally, the post office that sends goods and supplies out to all functions of the city, including pigmentation—the mysterious Golgi Apparatus!

The Eukaryotic Cells

This simple analogy has given the public and even physicians an easy and new way to think about the many functions of skin cells and how we can influence them topically from the outside in, as well as vice-versa. The question of course, is how do cells achieve all their functions in such a small, diverse and crowded space inside this tiny "city"?

The answer lies in the little talked about Eukaryotic cells. Like the Fascia, eukaryotic cells have vast dimension in the health and maintenance of the human body, including skin, yet are seldom mentioned in topical protocol—or product knowledge classes where the catch-all phrase of "skin care" can be as ambiguous as "well, it just works."

Eukaryotic cells partition off different functions in the main cell, rather like rooms in a house or an apartment. These specialized compartments are called organelles and play different roles within the cell.

The mitochondria generate energy for every other organelle in the skin via oxygen from the blood and from food molecules; lysosome enzymatically breakdown and recycle organelles and macromolecules. The endoplasmic reticulum helps to build new walls (membranes) and to transport proteins throughout the cell. All work together for a common cause, bound and assisted by the eukaryotic cells.

The membranes that surround eukaryotic organelles are based upon lipid bilayers and are like the cell's outer membrane "wall." Together the total area of the cell's integral membrane far exceeds that of the plasma membrane—just like the fascia far exceeds the skin or the epidermis as the body's largest organ (although technically not called an organ).

Of all the eukaryotic envelope that surrounds the nucleus and keeps the DNA from the cell's protein synthesis apparatus, tiny shunts (pores) in the envelope (called nuclear pores) determine which macromolecules can enter or exit the nucleus (which includes the messenger RNA that carry "requests" from the DNA to the protein manufacturing centers in the cytoplasm).

All this 24/7 activity takes milli-seconds to happen and can be influenced and maintained by the presence of co-enzymes (vitamins), essential amino acids, essential oils, thermogenics (heat), and cryogenics (cold) and, electromagnetic waves.

In addition, the DNA possesses memory banks that, due to poor skin maintenance, can go "dormant" rendering the skin premature demise. However, with circulation stimulation, pulse and rest-phase of the peripheral capillaries and the lymph nodes, the intricate mechanics of the eukaryotic organelles can function at top performance—which basically is maximum skin health.

Injectables and Fillers

New, popular fillers that "almost mock" our matrix is thought to be more or less benign (as opposed to fillers possessing various granules or so-called "nano particles"). And in truth, a good innocuous hyaluronic-based filler usually does not call upon any defense mechanisms of the skin, sort of ignoring the presence of a good "fake" that occupies a deflated area of the face or body where the matrix has thinned out over time, or adipose fat has shifted or been burned away by carbohydrate depravation.

Only in skin that has all eukaryotic organelles operating night and day at full capacity, do fillers have a chance to survive for any manageable length of time. Poorly functioning organelles and a faltering mitochondrion will perceive sugars in the glycoamino glycans, and salts in the hyaluronic acids, as nutrients—and quickly attempt to devour the filler.

Topical skin revision works with skin structure, pigmentation, and function—all successfully. Fillers, threads, and even cosmetic surgery become adjunctive to "fine tune" the good skin regeneration work, rather than "the main event" as commonly practiced in today's modern aesthetics.

The epidermis and everything underneath, always shifting and changing cell configuration, is a wonderful organic computer and laboratory with enormous memory capacity. But, like any complicated machine, it requires an "all-over tune up" and proper lubricants, energy—and in the human case, nutrient components—to regain its original functions and withstand environmental, hormonal and gravity assaults.

> The mind can control the health outcomes of many diseases, even cancer.

Holistic Vs. Wholistic

The word HOLISTIC has become popular again, but I prefer the term to WHOLISTIC, meaning "the entire body"—with each cell group interconnected and bound to the next group.

We are in age of precision now. A good example is what I witnessed in Riga, Latvia, at an aesthetic medical conference. There I saw the remarkable skills of German medical doctor, Sabine Zenker, as she demonstrated her very precise "mapping of the facial dimensions" before administering various fillers using a varieties of syringes to all levels of the patient's face and neck—including areas close to the bone. This pain-staking methodology is truly state-of-the-art: no quick fix here! With the vast amount of technology available today, by using the right chemistry, and a wholistic outside-in approach during our daily skin care practice, we can improve the skin, even repair it.

Think Health and Healthy Skin

The mind can control the health outcomes of many diseases, even cancer. The placebo effect is very real, as we are finding out. That said, the cells themselves must have the right chemistry that comes from outside sources (which is what the preface ESSENTIAL means) before the mind can take control. It is like driving a well-maintained car as opposed to one that has had little maintenance: which one drives the best and the longest?

12

Tight for a Night: Enzyme and Oxygen Therapy

Body skin, like facial skin, can lose elasticity over time. Persons who were sun worshipers in their younger years and persons who have been on yo-yo weight loss diets are especially prone to crepe-like or wrinkled, loose body skin. However, unlike the facial skin that is in direct contact with the facial muscles, body skin does not possess the same underlying dermal infrastructure. Hence even workouts and weight lifting, even on a regular basis, which may tone muscles will not tighten up the loose skin.

Fibroblast cells in the skin slow down collagen production. Elastin's are broken over large areas of tissue. With minimal collagen being produced and mass amounts of elastin fibers irrevocably broken, the skin loses turgidity and bounce. Likewise, dead cells build up on the surface as a defense mechanism, an armor plate as it were, against the assault of free radical and sun damage. These cells appear as crinkly or "chicken skin" and are especially obvious when the legs are crossed, or the skin is moved during certain body positions. It is during these positions when the skin looks most crepe-like and geriatric.

In these cases, the intercellular matrix has also thinned down over time, causing the skin to be more fragile and tissue paper looking! This is due to a lack of essential fatty acids. This also means that the GAGs (glycosaminoglycans) in the body skin have been compromised.

Enzyme Therapy

Nothing is ever permanently cured, but many skin conditions can be revised and maintained. The first step would be to remove the redundant cuticle build up, all those shiny, wrinkly-looking dead cells. Alpha Hydroxy Aid serums can be used in treatment to some degree, but then there is the irritation factor over time and the risk of acid hardened skin or skin that becomes over-thin and more susceptible to the sun's damage.

I have used low level acids and retinoids in professional treatment on a temporary basis for legs that were blotchy with small, milia-like bumps or various other dermatitis, but I have found that the best cuticle removal system for lose body skin is enzyme therapy.

A body enzyme treatment has been recently discovered that not only removes cuticle build-up on the skin via reverse osmosis but tightens and tones up sagging body skin and may last for twenty-four hours after the first treatment (hence the nickname "Tight for a Night!"). Subsequent treatments have longer lasting and maintainable results, but the main action in this treatment is brought about through a process I refer to as "Plasmatic Regeneration."

The blood to the skin (plasma) is offered through the capillary loops under the skin. Stimulating the valves of these loops increases oxygen from inside the body. The oxygen in turn stimulates the skin cell's power battery, an organelle called the Mitochondria. The Mitochondria then produces more energy giving and life promoting ATP (adenosinetriphospate) which is sort of the biological electricity for the body. Likewise, the increased oxygen removes toxins from the living cells—one of the functions of our blood in the first place!

For oxygen to benefit the body, it must first be breathed into the lungs, then stored in the alveoli until needed.

I have worked on clients who had cold, white flesh on their legs and have noticed that after a body enzyme treatment, their legs had more feeling, were rosy in color and much firmer in tensor. Spraying oxygen on the outside of the skin or applying so-called oxygen cremes (cremes made with peroxide) on the skin will NOT increase the oxygen in the capillary loops and will in fact, damage the skin cells—which is why we have Antioxidants.

For oxygen to benefit the body, it must first be breathed into the lungs, then stored in the alveoli until needed. For bodies getting older, it is important to force the oxygen to leave the alveoli and empty into the veins where it becomes bonded with hemoglobin. This in turn goes into the capillaries and is ultimately deposited into the mitochondria. On the return trip, it takes toxins away from the cells.

Oxygen Therapy

Oxygen therapy is once again popular (I have survived three revivals of it over the last thirty odd years) but in physiology, these are what they really are and all the buzz words or pseudo-scientific theories in the world cannot change how the body really works and what it responds to. There is an enormous amount of real medical and scientific data on the body and oxygen that opposes the popular theory of topically applied oxygen. We also discovered in our research that the hydrolysis of dead and dying skin cells and the increase of circulation in the skin is not quite enough. We observed that after the remarkable body enzyme treatments and after all the old cuticle was removed, the living cells left behind needed nutritional support to keep them alive longer.

Delivery of these nutrients had to be devised for the body enzyme to become a true, anti-aging treatment. This is where TRANSDERMAL CREMES come into the picture. Cremes made of plant proteins, transdermal formulated (a long, costly process, not popular with most laboratories) can deliver all the vitamins, minerals and proteins needed to keep a living skin cell alive longer.

After removing the body enzyme, a tedious and messy process for the therapist, we learned to spray the body with an herb and mineral based water and then massage our transdermal creme into the skin while it was still wet from the water. The tightening and firming of legs, derrieres and tummies was amazing and often lasted several days.

Evening Primrose

The body enzyme treatments just described are only half of the picture, however. The best topical treatment in the world is only partially effective if the client's intercellular matrix has thinned out with time, sun damage and stress. This matrix is what all the cells float in—a sort of jelly-like substance made of hyaluronic acids with its salts and other GAGs, all kept hydrated by the chondroïtine (such as citric acid). We are describing a gel cleverly put together by Nature using salts, sugars and fats! All protein structures involving the skin are held in place by this gel. If it becomes too thin, dermal hydration is lost and the turgidity and bounce to the skin dissipates.

The only way to strengthen this matrix and thicken it up

again is to take Essential Fatty Acids (EFAs) internally. There are various types of EFAs on the market that range from fish sources, flax seed oils to borage oils, and oils too exotic and too expensive to be of practical, daily use. All these oils offer some Omega 3 and Omega 6 EFAs, but none can be compared to the incredible oil extracted from a simple plant (a weed, really), the Evening Primrose.

Not only does 100% pure Evening Primrose Oil (EPO) help to increase the essential fatty acids in the skin, thus thickening thin and crepe-like skin back to its youthful "bounce," but it helps to regulate hormonal problems, reverse and inhibit sun damage, clear up chronic eczema and psoriasis and other dermatitis and even assists in clearing acne. Evening Primrose also contains a great deal of tocopherol (vitamin E) which is our primary anti-oxidant source.

> 100% pure Evening Primrose Oil (EPO) help to increase the essential fatty acids in the skin, thus thickening thin and crepe-like skin back to its youthful "bounce," but it helps to regulate hormonal problems, reverse and inhibit sun damage, clear up chronic eczema and psoriasis and other dermatitis and even assists in clearing acne.

A good amount of the Evening Primrose Oil we see in the health food stores comes from China. While there is nothing wrong with plants being grown in China, the process of extraction used by many Chinese herbal companies dilutes or erodes the full power of the Evening Primrose Oil. Most of this is done by the cold press method which really does not cold press the tiny pips from the Evening Primrose at all. These pips are so small that when they are run through the cold press machine, the machine increases its revolutions to a high speed to extract the oil. This friction heats the oil, hence a large percentage of its powers are removed.

Fortunately, Australia has come to our rescue! An English botanist (retired in New Zealand after working for big pharmaceutical companies for years) had in his possession an exclusive Hexane method for extracting the oil from the Evening Primrose. Remarkably, it had maintained its purity and 100% of all its incredible powers and energy.

The Canterbury plains in New Zealand are known for their rich, volcanic soils and high mineral content flowing down from the surrounding mountain's snow melt. We found Evening Primrose growing there at a ranch that provided the botanist a wonderful source from which he could extract the oil. I and hundreds of others in the last year have taken internally this Evening Primrose extract from this exclusive source. I have noticed, amongst other things, that the skin on the backs of my hands was becoming smoother and thicker, more like my hands were at age 30! Others have noticed the cutaneous tissue on various parts of their bodies reacting the same way. The obvious EPO benefits from eczema, psoriasis and hormonally imbalance persons have been manifested, as well.

We feel very fortunate that this little paradise called New Zealand came up with an internal answer to aging body skin to complement our many years of research on topical body treatments. It was a New Zealand therapist, Alex Proctor, who together with N. Zed Beauty and Consumer advocate Florence Barret, brought to our attention the importance of the intercellular matrix in the first place.

Ms. Barrett tried to get me interested in this subject whilst attending a press conference I was conducting in Hong Kong nearly ten years ago. Her theories were manifested by Mrs. Alex Clark (then Proctor) in dozens of practical treatments, with so many terrific results that our international research team went searching for a dependable and pure form of EPO.

That we would find it in New Zealand, brought the whole scientific venture into a full circle.

13

Body Treatments: Treating Cellulite and Loose Skin

Cellulite is a term for lumpy, dimpled flesh on the thighs, hips, buttocks and abdomen. It's most common in adolescent and adult women. Although not a serious medical condition, many who have it, detest it, and are embarrassed by it.

Cellulite looks like dimpled or bumpy skin. It's sometimes described as having a cottage cheese or orange peel texture. You can see mild cellulite only if you pinch your skin in an area where you have cellulite, such as your thighs. More severe cellulite makes the skin appear rumpled and bumpy with areas of peaks and valleys.

Cellulite is most common around the thighs and buttocks, but it can be found on the breasts, lower abdomen and upper arms as well.

Cellulite isn't a serious medical condition, and treatment isn't necessary. In fact, many doctors consider cellulite a normal occurrence.

Little is known about what causes cellulite, but it involves fibrous connective cords that tether the skin to the underlying muscle, with the fat lying between. As fat cells accumulate, they push up against the skin, while the long, tough cords pull down. This creates an uneven surface or dimpling.

Cellulite is much more common in women than in men, but men can have it, too. In fact, most women develop some cellulite after puberty. This is because women's fat is typically distributed in the thighs, hips and buttocks—common areas for cellulite. Cellulite is also more common with aging, when the skin loses elasticity.

Some common causes of cellulite:
- Weight gain can make cellulite more noticeable, but some lean people have cellulite, as well.
- Cellulite tends to run in families, so genetics might play the biggest role in whether you develop cellulite.
- An inactive lifestyle also can increase your chances of having cellulite.

- Pregnancy can cause cellulite.

Treatments to Minimize the Appearance of Cellulite

Many cellulite treatments, including massages or cellulite creams, advertise great results, but most of these treatments don't live up to their claims. While researchers are studying possible medical treatments, until and unless some magical pill or treatment comes along, there are things you can do to slightly improve the appearance of cellulite.

The three-wrinkle cleavage and bat wing arms comes to everyone no matter how much muscle tone or fat sculpting one does. It can only by eradicated by Body Enzyme Treatments with its dead cells removal, reverse osmosis homeostasis action, deep plasmatic effect on the mitochondria, and actual tissue lifting effects—simply by "waking up" all the cellular systems that was present in our skins in the first place.

Cellulite, "muffin-top" waist lines (or spare tires for men), while at times bulging dimpled thighs, and flabby, puffy arms, have been the bane of humanity for years. Excess and abundant flesh was popular such as depicted in paintings of classic artist Sir Peter Paul Rubens in the 16th century as well as sign of wealth in culture other periods, those days are largely in the past. Today our understanding is that obesity is not healthy and of course, almost any sign fat deposits are to some completely unacceptable. Hence, liposuction is in. **Liposuction** does not remove cellulite unless it is accompanied by skin tightening surgery such as the tummy tuck. Seaweed or herbal wraps also do nothing to remove cellulite.

Cellulite can be temporarily removed—and maintained. Here are some of the best ways to do that.

Massage. Without a doubt, massage therapy has many physiological benefits that extend far beyond mere relaxation. So much so that at the decades famous Baden-Baden spa in Germany, each massage practitioner must have a medical certification to be employed. Our "medi-spas" are somewhat different. Certainly, we have access to top massage therapists, physiotherapists and reflexologists. The "medi" in medi spa has nothing to do however with these experts. It is usually Doctors (GPs, Podiatrists and occasionally a dermatologist) coming in by appointment only to administer BOTOX®, fillers or other injectables, including approved micro-needling. Sometimes a physician will have ownership in the spa and have his or her practice next door or in the same facility. Nothing wrong with this, in fact, it's ideal and DMK International has been doing this for many years overseas.

It's the spa treatments themselves that are somewhat lacking. Real results in revising body skin and other anomalies will not be achieved with Jacuzzis, infra-red saunas, smothering people in herbal slime then wrapping them in a foil sheet or covering them with hot rocks. While all these common practices are relaxing (and in the case of infra-red sauna, skin detoxification does take place but only at the epidermal level), fundamental changes in loose, saggy skin, muffin tops, back boobs and rough, hyperpigmented decollates do not happen.

Why shouldn't the body tissue also have such dramatic results? It can. But let's examine a few common body problems and how they respond to the right treatment and home regimen. If these principles are taken seriously, the entire Spa industry would change.

What is Cellulite?

Cellulite is medically categorized into 4 stages:
1. Alterations to the pre-capillary system leading to subtle changes in vascular permeability which in turn leads to interadipositary transudation (edema);
2. Edema causes metabolic changes that become hyperplasia and hypertrophy of the reticular network;
3. At this "round-robin" point (takes several cycles of repetition) collagen fibers organize around groups of white adipose fat cells forming micronodules; and,
4. A union of these micronodules form macro nodules that create cellulite.

There are basically three manifestations of cellulite:
✓ Saggy "mattress-like" skin with several depressions or dimples and some elevations, created by the irregular retraction of the skin;
✓ Orange peel look due to the tumefaction of the skin and dilation of the follicular pores; and,
✓ A very dimpled "cottage cheese" appearance of the skin in affected areas including under upper arms, sometimes accompanied by the "bat wing" effect.

Almost all women and a few men have had some form of cellulite in their lives—and detest it! Many have tried the roll-and-suck machines resembling a huge praying mantis, or the old G5 battering ram machine (both can be very damaging to the vascular and fascia of the body) and a variety of wet, herbal wraps. A lot of these are booked on day 2 of a summer cruise to look good on the decks or by the pool.

The "muffin top" waist syndrome that plague males are also another treatment area that keeps a man religious with his diet and gym or other workouts because he can see and feel a result in that area after the first measurable treatment!

"Fixing" Cellulite

Some of this surface trauma can be partially eliminated with surgery including implants, as loose tissue appears tighter as excess is cut away. But many are not candidates for this due to down time, expense or other physical limitations. Over the last 45 years, I have learned that all cases of cellulite can be controlled by three modalities, each working in tandem with the other.

Thermogenic or "Pseudo Heat"

The first way to control cellulite is with thermogenic or "pseudo heat" (chemical heat as opposed to Celsius). Plants that yield rubescent or volatile oils that stimulate the ganglia in the skin with a heat sensation change the shape of the hardened, toxic white adipose fat cells in the tissue that is lumpy with depressions and elevations. The hard cells smooth out and match the normal fat cells, the skin appearing less "cottage cheese." Think of placing a stick of butter from the refrigerator on a hot stove. The butter-fat is changed from a solid state to a liquid oil state. Same action.

Formulas compounded by water-into-oil cremes or lotions (old school, expensive but very trans-epidermal) can be stored in the skin, using plastic wraps to hold it in place for up to an hour. The non-porosity of the plastic keeps bouncing the thermogenic effect into the hard-fat cells over and over until they finally give up and change shape.

Accurate measurements are a must in this type of treatment to give a record of how many inches are lost each treatment. There is always an inch loss if performed properly with the right formulations. It will not work on bulky muscle tissue, however.

Cryotherapy and Ultra Sound

Cryotherapy is the opposite modality, using the "cold method" to push excess fluids away from fatty tissue in cases of edematous cellulite (soft and puffy cellulite). The current medical Cool SCULPTING was based on this principle, although advertisements claim your fat is frozen then hydrolyzed away. Not quite scientific but it sounds good! Either way the results are the same on the appropriate cellulite category—except one is much less expensive and does not require an MD.

Ultrasound is added to cryotherapy. I have seen great results when ultrasound is added to cryotherapy; you can mix the conducting gel 50/50 with your cryo gel (if it has no salts in it as a conductor). I created a well-known topical analgesic for pain many years ago, called BIOFREEZE™, and after I sold out my interest to big pharma I experimented with the formula for cellulite and was surprised at the ongoing results.

I had to make changes for cellulite work since the original formula for pain management was far too harsh for cellulite treatments. Deep Freeze Therapy products, made by a Texas sports pain management company, is ideal for body treatments.

LED Red and Infrared

LED red and infrared research has shown some promising results on all types of cellulite. Within the deeper dermis, there have been results in modulations in cell functions, cell proliferations and the repair of compromised cells. Synthesis of ATP in the mitochondria, mRNA, and reverse transcriptase polymerase change reactions, collagen and elastic production, increased levels of tissue matrix, and induced mitosis or aptosis can all be modulated, initiated or even inhibited by LED energy from one or more wave lengths.

It's difficult to choose machines now days that rely on popularity of device, bells and whistles, but dodgy performance and little back up or guarantees. I have found that it takes a combination of modalities to get a great body treatment result.

As human beings, at our most simplified denominator, we are a bag of fluids, a few chemicals, orchestrated by enzymes and held together with electromagnetic waves! Every chemical action in our cell regulation has an enzyme involved at some point. Enzymes are part of bad reactions, as well as the good ones. Which ones to employ in positive therapy and which ones to negate already in the cells, has been my life-long quest. It's a truly fascinating field.

14

The Truth about Glycolic Acid

Gycolic acid is a colorless, translucent, crystalline compound, $C_2H_4O_3$, that occurs in cane sugar, unripe grapes, and sugar beets and has numerous industrial uses, especially in dyeing leather and textiles and in the manufacture of pesticides. It reacts with the top layer of skin, breaking it down by dissolving sebum and other substances that bind cells together. Made up of small molecules, it is able to penetrate the skin deeply and easily. This makes it most effective for treating fine lines, acne, blackheads, dullness, oiliness and uneven texture. Dead skin cells are sloughed off revealing smoother, brighter, younger looking skin. The products available which feature Glycolic Acid range in percentage of concentration.

One of the most overrated ingredients in skin products is glycolic acid, but before you throw out any product, here are the facts garnered from clinical test trials and manufacturers who are impartial to cosmetic company opinions or claims being made in the market place.

Glycolic Acid is no different from any other synthetic or natural chemical in that it is available in a variety of grades or purities, depending on its intended use. Once we only had two grades available: reagent and technical (industrial grade), both encompassing the two extremes on the purity scale. Now we have a confusing array of purity grades that include ACS, reagent, CP (chemically pure), USP (US Pharmacopoeia Specifications), NF (National Formulary Specifications), food grade, feed grade, ratio grade, semiconductor grade, research grade (my favorite), spectro grade, chemical grade, commercial grade, injectable grade, nitration grade, and tech grade (industrial). Whew!

In between all of these "purity" grades are the new designer formulas that allow a skin-care manufacturing company to advertise their glycolic products as "special" or more advanced. But here's the thing: Glycolic acid is just glycolic acid, and purity is not really that important to the glycolic acid peel procedure itself, because even the lowest industrial grades of glycolic are not the heavy, toxic metal types found in other chemicals.

What is more of concern is the presence of formic acid and sulfates found in higher strength, technical grade glycolics, which make this grade of acid more unpredictable than glycolic acids listed under cosmetic grade. However, most glycolics are formulated in strengths that easily and safely accommodate any impurities from cosmetic grade down to technical grade (5-10% strength in a crème base applied to a layer of dead skin cells).

There is no need to worry about the new designer glycolic acids that claim to go beyond cosmetic grade in purity, this is like comparing tap water to brook water, technical grade being the brook water. The purveyors of the new glycolic acids, many of them medical doctors, are aware of the potential enormous profits to be made in the Beauty Therapy Field and are claiming to have better glycolic than ever before. You will see advertisements that scream about the benefits of "Super Buffered-Time-Release" glycolic acid or "Acetyl/Catalyzed" glycolic acid (this one is very misleading, even to a professional chemist).

These so called medically designed glycolic acid for the aesthetician are not mentioned in any chemical reference index or in any raw material listings from chemical and pharmaceutical supply houses, anywhere. In fact, they are compounded formulas containing glycolic acid.

There is no secret special laboratory somewhere where a doctor is mass producing "special, super charged glycolic acids."

Understanding Glycolic Acid

The terms such as "Acetyl/Catalyzed" or "Buffered-Time-Release" are describing a PROCESS used in formulating the product, not some special or superior type of glycolic acid. But the advertising of such products is very misleading especially when the ads say, "Our products are beyond the twenty-first century of ordinary Glycolics" or "The next generation of Glycolic Acids!" Usually these ads include realistic graphs and charts showing how their product performs better than the regular glycolic acid. What the message does NOT say is that their products contain the same grade of glycolic acid that is available to any cosmetic company. There is no secret special laboratory somewhere where a doctor is mass producing "special, super charged glycolic acids."

Another controversy involving terms used in the marketing of glycolic acid is the references to the strengths and "sharpness" of the acid. Non-chemists have loosely applied chemical terms to their products. Again, this makes it more difficult for the therapist to determine the key ingredient.

Here are some of the more common terms used.

Neutralized Glycolic Acid: This process involves a salt whose name has no reference to the name glycolic acid. What is questionable is whether this salt has any physical benefit to the skin. Buffered and Stabilized glycolics are even more confusing as to what chemical claims are being made! When you shield glycolic acid from its innate peeling action, you are also shielding the effective peeling action from the skin. This means more frequent applications, thus more trauma to the skin in the long run. Another example to illustrate this would be that of a hairdresser trying to bleach virgin black hair to platinum blond using a mild 20% volume peroxide with the bleach. This combination must be applied to the hair 3-4 times to achieve maximum blondness, as opposed to a quick bleach using 60% peroxide. The weaker bleach destroys the hair each time it is applied. Stronger bleach lifts out color very quickly, preserving the integrity of the hair.

The skin reacts much the same with buffered or stabilized glycolic acids, so there is the all-important question, "Are buffered or stabilized 10% glycolic acids any more effective or any less risky than a well formulated 4% straight glycolic?"

The answer is that lower level strength, straight glycolic well blended with other AHAs is much more effective and gives better results over time.

Glycol Polymers and Lactolpolymers: Other alternatives to using straight glycolic acid in formulas are the Polymer forms of AHAs such as glycol polymers and lactolpolymers. The claim for these polymers is that they are "smarter" than other AHAs because of their shorter oligomer chain formations. These molecules allegedly align themselves naturally with the skin's own keratolytic pathways, thus lessening the disruption of surrounding structures.

I have found this type of free acid is more random in effects and less predictable than other types of AHAs, but ideal for "spot" work such as heavy etched wrinkles around the mouth. I do not recommend polymerized AHAs for all-over facial application.

In the final analysis, technique and the application of products can be more important than products themselves.

Combinations: The unfortunate aspect of glycolic acid products is that they are popularly believed to be a "cure all" for every situation ranging from fine lines and wrinkles, to severe acne vulgaris. However, there are special conditions of the skin that do not respond well to a sudden lowering of the skin's pH to around 3.1 (which is the pH of most AHA solutions that work). This would include those who have extremely dehydrated skins, since AHAs work off available moisture in the skin, even down to the bilayer fluids with constant, everyday usage.

Another type of skin condition not a candidate for AHA therapy would be folliculitis, or any other acne condition accompanied by superfluous hair (hirsute). Those who have a combination of aging skin, acne, acne scars, and excess facial hair, all at the same time. Glycolic acid products simply would not address all these related disorders effectively. You would need a COMBINATION of treatments, each with a different type of chemical action but all working towards the common goal of smooth, healthy skin.

Raising the pH with Alkalis

There are products that start out in a dry, powder form that become very alkaline when mixed with herbal water into a smooth paste. Basically, thioglycolic depilatories, these products will raise the pH of the skin to nearly 10 on the pH scale in less than four minutes. Facial hair dissolves instantly, the hair follicle is completely de-congested as skin cells that plug it up along with old, hardened sebum wax are rendered completely squamous. Literally everything on the skin's surface is softened so quickly that all the dead protein is easily flushed away. Pustules that have hardened into cystic acne open without squeezing or extractions, and in-grown hairs disappear before your eyes.

After the treatment, the therapist restores the pH of the

skin back to normal with a natural neutralizing lotion. After a few days of resting the skin, the client can then have an AHA treatment to remove the rest of the dead skin cells on other areas of the face or body that are not affected by folliculitis. However, many times after this Alkaline based treatment, AHA products are not necessary.

For aging clients with hyperpigmentation, we find that a combination of Enzyme treatments to hydrolyze impurities from the skin and tighten it up, followed by a quick peeling, low strength phenol acid in a natural gel base, not only removes fine line and wrinkles, but strengthens the underlying tissues. It also prepares the skin for more advanced pigmentation products, such as azelaic acid, kojic acid, and oleic acid formulations.

Alkalizing the site of hyperpigmentation (such as melasma, chloasma) before applying the pigmentation removing products is a far better way to ensure maximum penetration than "acidifying" the area with glycolic acid. Purging the dark pigmentation areas with ice after alkalizing the skin also ensures rapid removal of the excess melanin. Many manufactures have made the mistake of adding AHAs to their pigmentation removal creams and lotions, even products containing hydroquinone, in the mistaken belief that AHAs will make the pigmentation destroying ingredients penetrate faster. In fact, adding AHAs to such a formula may only increase trauma to the skin over the long run, and trauma contributes to hyperpigmentation!

Do not believe that one single miracle ingredient such as glycolic acid is the panacea of all disorders, regardless of what form it may come in! And do not be misled into believing there are superior glycolic acids coming in the market; glycolic acid is what it is.

Safe Home Products with AHAs

Body Lotions containing more than 10% total strength of combination AHAs. Apply to cleansed skin once a week before soaking in a hot tub (leave on 15-20 minutes before tub bathing or shower). A neat solution of AHA, 10% in strength, applied locally to pimples or pustules on the body and left overnight will usually remove the blemishes within hours.

Unsafe AHA Home Products

- Facial cremes containing any amount of AHA used daily.

- Shampoos containing AHAs in any strength, especially on permed hair. AHA shampoos will weaken the perm or break off permed hair immediately. This also applies to chemically straightened hair.

- Sunblock's containing AHAs. The sun traumatizes the skin with radiation, why add extra trauma to the skin and excite the defense systems, like promoting excess pigmentation?

In the final analysis, technique and the application of products can be more important than products themselves.

15

The Enzymatic Body: Enzyme Therapy and Skin Treatments

I have been called the Enzyme King by the press due to my research on the subject, and yet after 50 years I feel that I am just at the tip of a very large iceberg.

Enzymes themselves are the Kings because they rule over every organism on this planet. In the modern world of "quick fixes" which include skin fillers, BOTOX®, surgical threads, and all kinds of radio frequency, and laser machines, if I were asked to select ONE treatment that in the long term gives the best results, I would have to say Enzyme Therapy. In China, for example, where most skins are not suitable for lasers and some other treatments, enzyme therapy can not only restore the cellular functions of youth and tighten sagging contours, but is the first step in the removal and total control of hyperpigmentation.

If we ask our top scientists to describe the human body at its fundamental level, the scientist would have to conclude (as you hear me repeat in this book) *"The human being is primarily a bag of fluids, proteins and amino acids, orchestrated by enzymes and held together by electromagnetic energy!"*

Science has identified only 1300 enzymes that control every molecular aspect of our bodies, and I am convinced there are many more. It is not surprising to me that enzymes play an important role in the treatment of the disorders of the skin. After all, it is a series of enzymatic activities that maintain the skin at its healthiest in the first place.

> Enzymes rule over every organism on this planet.

Anatomy of an Enzyme

Enzymes are nature's biological catalysts. It was commonly believed by skin therapists and even physicians, that enzymes were not suitable for real skin therapy because they were huge, protein molecules—too big to penetrate the skin. The fact is, enzymes are not proteins any more than a light bulb is electricity. Skin therapy enzymes USE proteins formed in plant cells to act as organic catalysts in initiating or speeding up specific chemical reactions.

Research shows that enzymes combine temporarily with the reacting molecule. Mutual contact of surrounding molecules is then no longer a matter of chance, but a matter of certainty. Hence a faster reaction. As an example, when the body breaks down a carbohydrate, the energy used to hold the carbohydrate is released and immediately used or stored in the body. This is called "metabolism." **Metabolism** is divided into two functions: anabolism (for synthesis of cell material) and catabolism (for the decomposition of cell material).

These reactions would be very slow unless assisted by proteins orchestrated by enzymes. Without enzymes the entire concept of metabolic function would be lost.

Enzymes work by joining to the substrate (reactant) to form an enzyme-substrate complex and then produce the products of the reaction.

The enzyme itself never changes and is not used up in this reaction but is released for repeated use. Think of an enzyme as a space station in outer space. Around this station could be many different types of space ships flying at random, not interacting with each other at all, thus accomplishing no missions. Each space station has a docking port for a specific style of space ship. If the ship docks in its own port and another ship lands in its correct place on the space station, they are held in "stasis" and can interact with each other and then things happen. This is how an enzyme works.

Enzymes and Skin Revision Treatments

There are many enzyme and coenzyme (vitamin) activities in the skin that regulate its normal functions. For example, the enzyme collagenase helps to regulate the synthesis of collagen fibers. If collagenase is destroyed by invasion of an aggressive treatment, such as the drug Ro-Accutane (normally given to acne patients), the collagen fibers rush to any source of trauma to the skin such as laser resurfacing or acid peels. The result may be a keloid or **hypertrophic scar**. This is one of the reasons the old-time phenol acid or trichloroacetic acid peels left the patient's skin looking plastic or waxy. The NORMAL proliferation of collagen fibers was accelerated and rushed to the surface to participate in repair and remodeling of the skin too quickly.

However, there are many enzymes that can be applied topically to the skin that are extremely beneficial. They can assist in removing the buildup of dead skin cells (often misdiagnosed as "dry skin") that manifest in superficial wrinkles.

Enzymes can also release gases, impurities and other effluvia from the skin, as well. This type of treatment can result in a younger and tighter skin. It is not a case of "how many enzymes are used in formulation" to accomplish this, but rather, the stimulation of enzyme activity in the skin itself. If the correct formulations of enzymes are applied to the skin, hydrolysis of the dead cells and the impurities burdening the living cells begins in about twenty minutes.

Topically Applied Enzymes

Enzymes are categorized into several groups. Some dissolve dead protein, others digest starches and excess glucose. Still others help to break up solidified oils in the shunts or openings of the skin. A special enzyme, transferase, can send messages across cell membranes. This is called "Transcription."

In this process, a strand of messenger RNA is synthesized according to the nitrogenous base code of DNA. The Enzyme RNA polymerase binds to one of the DNA molecules in the double helix. The other strand remains dormant. RNA moves along the DNA strand reading the nucleotides one by one. The enzyme selects complementary bases from available nucleotides and positions them in an mRNA molecule according to the principle of complimentary base pairing. The mRNA molecule then carries the genetic message to the cytoplasm for protein synthesis.

This is vital information for all skin cells as well to keep them alive longer and healthier—while removing the burden of the dead cuticle. Dead cuticle is the buildup of dead skin cells over a lifetime that helps to create dry, wrinkled and uneven toned skin.

Living Enzymes: What Enzymes Eat

Years ago, I discovered that the best base to store inert, yet still living enzymes, was in the zygote base Albumin. Albumin is from the inside membrane of egg shells and makes an ideal storage place for live enzymes that deactivate once exposed to aqueous fluids and air in about 45 to 60 minutes. In addition, I add lysozyme and Amylase. Amylase initiates the hydrolysis of glycoside linkages, part of the so-called "cellular glue" that helps bind dead cells to the underlying living cell stratum.

The starch-eating enzyme, Agrozyme, is also part of the formulation, as well as Grozyme, Rapidase and Superclastase. These enzymes are used for the treatment of sewage and human waste products. These are especially vital in the treatment of acne skin conditions.

Lipase is another "message carrying" enzyme that deals with lipids and fats in the skin and in addition to the above-mentioned enzymes I add the following components:

- **Aspartic Acid:** a roborant strengthens the tissues;

- **Lysine:** an amino acid that improves protein quality in tissue and is one of the three amino acids necessary for collagen production;

- **Proline and Glycine:** the other two amino acids in collagen production, are energized into action by vitamin C. Glycine is also anti-pruritic (anti-itch) which is of great benefit to eczema type skin conditions;

- **Lecithin:** rich in linoleic acid; and,

- **Copper Chlorophyll:** promotes healing and photosynthesis of any active botanical used in formulation.

Other enzyme treatments bring about a "plasmatic action" in the skin by dilating all the peripheral capillaries. This brings about improved oxygen uptake from INSIDE the body. This increased oxygen is deposited in the correct amounts into the mitochondria, which requires oxygen to produce enough ATP for anti-aging results. You can literally see this effect on the skin of the neck, face and decollate following an enzyme treatment. There is very little, if any, superficial erythema, but the capillaries stand out like a road map, proving the effects of the enzyme's treatment goes deep enough for total dilation of the peripheral capillaries.

This is true oxygen therapy as opposed to the dangers or

lack of positive results from applying oxygen cremes (merely peroxide) or spraying the skin with compressed oxygen.

Facial Muscles and Enzymes

The fragile, underlying facial muscles can be pumped up to a stronger level much as any muscle in the body can with regular weight training and exercise. However, facial exercises are tedious and require a religious daily routine to achieve and maintain results. Most of us will not devote the appropriate time to this type of a regimen. Electrical stimulation with the so-called face-lift machines offers only about a 20% result in muscle stimulation. Research of this modality has shown that treatment every day using specific micro-current results in the 20% muscle increase and must be maintained nearly daily.

It's a rigorous process, and few achieve such devotion! Voluntary contraction of facial muscles using enzyme treatments has a much more natural and lasting effect as the muscles themselves are moving on their own accord against resistance. This is also known as **isometric exercise**. In a voluntary reaction of a muscle, there is an asynchronous firing of motor neurons in a smooth contraction. The more units that are involved, the further increase of muscle force being achieved.

If you apply very strong enzyme "bands" to the skin from motor control point to motor control point, you can accomplish this voluntary action. Most facial, neck and decollate muscles are lateral, horizontal or vertical. These can be worked with predicable results. The oris oculi and oris orbicularis (muscles of the mouth and eyes) however, should not be treated in this manner, as they are round and unpredictable as to the direction they may contract.

Meat-Eating Enzymes

There are three crude enzymes commonly used in skin therapy for many years. Of all groups, these are the most aggressive as far as sensitizing the skin. These types of enzymes are also used in ordinary cooking in several countries under the label "Meat Tenderizers." Once sprinkled on a tough piece of meat, they will soften the meat almost to the point of desquamation in a few hours.

Likewise, if applied to the skin more than 15 minutes, they

will irritate the skin and the mucous membranes of the mouth, nose and eyes. These are bromelain (pineapple source) and papain (Papaya source). I use these only in cases of very thick, greasy type skins that have a lot of congestion and thick, dead cell build up.

Probably the best feature of enzyme therapy is that it has no real pH factor, either extremely acid or extremely alkaline. Therefore, contraindications are must less prevalent and/ or severe. But enzyme therapy formulation is not an easy process from the manufacturing level. It can be costly and time consuming in production. This alone does not make it attractive to most manufacturers of skin treatment products. I have depended upon the art of enzyme therapy as my primary form of skin revision and find its uses to be applicable in nearly every skin disorder or aging skin situation.

Enzymes and Lymph Drainage

The Doctor Voddar method of Lymph Drainage has been an acceptable form of detoxification therapy internationally for many years. Many American therapists are under the impression that lymph drainage therapy is accomplished with broad, sweeping massage movements from the lymph node areas of the neck down to the clavicle or breastbone.

The true application in fact, is a very precisely timed series of minute "pumping" manipulations that can be performed anywhere on the body. Elizabeth Stenvik of Trondheim, Norway, one of Northern Europe's top research therapists and a teacher of the Voddar method, is absolutely convinced that the Enzyme Muscle Contraction Therapy is another high-tech approach to lymph drainage. She has researched this potential in a series of in-clinic test trials and the results look promising.

This would explain why clients who undergo enzyme therapy have a much clearer, brighter and better-toned skin for many days following the treatment.

Reverse Osmosis and the Plasmatic Effect

There is no treatment in the world to date that can come close to comparing the homeostasis brought about by the DMK Enzyme Therapies. During the time period of 45 minutes a client is under DMK Masques One, Two and Three, many activities take place, the first being reverses osmosis in which fluids are forced through the cell wall membrane into the matrix, removing impurities and other effluvia. This leaves a nice clean cell and surrounding matrix.

After the initial application of enzyme masques, the client will experience sensations such as itching and then a regular pulsing as their own body temperature helps activate the enzymatic action on and within the skin. There will be a subtle dilation of all the peripheral capillaries, obvious on the client's skin after the masques are removed (normally disappearing after a few minutes.)

Many clients may be alarmed at this and assume it will create "broken capillaries." On the contrary, this action referred to as "plasmatic action" will not only flush out clogged capillaries that are viewed on the skin many times as "broken" but are in fact like mini-aneurisms ABOUT to break, but will strengthen the veins which are the very conduits of oxygen and nutrients that are taken up by the mitochondria, the "battery packs" that keep healthy skin cells alive.

It is this "road map" of capillaries that indicate a successful treatment and the assurance that the extra cellular fluids surrounding the cells are equalized. Extra cellular fluids that are too low or too high are indicated in skin that is unhealthy, inflamed or toxic. The DMK Enzyme treatments create the homeostasis (balanced extracellular fluids) that is necessary for healthy functioning skin.

It is the preservation of the mitochondria, the most important organelle in the skin cells that makes DMK treatments stand out as superior from any treatment offered in the market today.

16

The "PC Skin Disorder": The Effect of Electromagnetic Waves on Skin

Back in the late 1980s, the Norwegian Works League was researching a strange, rash-like effect, almost rosacea-like, appearing on people who were operating computers for long periods of time and especially those who were working in enclosed offices or spaces.

I had published a few articles on the incredible powers of controlled EMPW (electromagnetic pulsed waves) in relation to re-polarized damaged tissue, and stress related inflammation, as it related to cells becoming depolarized by an overload of the positive ion "throw away" electromagnetic waves coming off cell phones, televisions, and other electrical appliances.

The Norwegians, reading these articles, asked me to contribute to their research. At DMK International, we designed protocol that combated this disorder and called the condition "PC Skin."

At the time, I was concentrating on another epidemic, a sudden flurry of hyperpigmentation in Asia and Oriental countries whose deeper toned peoples are normally and naturally protected from sun damage. But after a recent meeting with the heads of SINTEF/Extreme Work Environment Bureau of Norway, I was convinced that both outbreaks were somewhat related.

The Institute of Physics, University of Oslo, and the Department of Dermatology regional Hospital, Trondheim, Norway, have been conducting a series of tests to support a growing suspicion that a lot of trauma to the skin is being perpetrated by electromagnetic waves.

Electromagnetic Waves (EMW)

Some people working with computers experience health problems that could be associated with both electric and electromagnetic fields. In my opinion, the fault lies mainly with the electromagnetic fields emitted by computers. Although the fields or waves are minimal and can barely be measured by an oscilloscope (therefore presumed "safe" by manufacturers), day-by-day exposure creates a sort of "build-up" of POSITIVE electromagnetic charge that has a domino or "knock-on" effect to the skin cells.

Most common symptoms are a sensation of burning, itching, prickling, stinging, and tightness. Other reports of redness, swelling and rashes have been coming in as well. Although these symptoms are less pronounced when screen filters are used to block most of the ELECTRIC fields, skin disorders persist—which leads me to believe that the electromagnetic waves are the culprit.

At DMK International, we have used this incredible force of nature in our treatments for many years, using properly manufactured EMW machines that emit pulsing waves from 100 to 1000 pulses per minute, passing through a bare skin contact antenna. Not only does this remove all stress from the client on contact, which is associated with acne and aging, but repolarizes all traumatized cells, as well.

Most of our active enzyme treatments are enhanced 100% when used in combination with EMWs. Collagen proliferation is also increased several times. With all these benefits from EMW's, why should they contribute to "PC skin"?

Throw-Away Waves

To better understand the function of EMWs in the human body, we must first examine the relationship of the brain to the other body parts. Think of the brain as a central computer, sending messages down conduits to each cell of the body, including skin cells. These communications are in the form of a NEGATIVE charge that go to the POSITIVE surface of cells and depolarize them, in other words, keeping the cells functioning normally.

The cell wall is also maintained by two chemicals, sodium and potassium. This is medically referred to as the Sodium Potassium Pump. The negative charge from the brain, which is part of the natural electromagnetic field of the body, helps cells taking valuable potassium to EXPEL sodium.

If, by some chance, this communication from the brain is interrupted, the POSITIVE charged surface of the cells takes over and expels the potassium, taking in sodium, and the cell goes into trauma. Inflammation, Oedema, and a whole host of invasive bacteria and viruses can then come into the open door of the cell. Therefore, successful electromagnetic therapy requires UNIPOLARITY, positive/negative charge moving through the body simultaneously. When there is a breakdown in communication and the cells go into trauma, applying the EMW machine that emits very low energy will repolarize the damaged cell in about thirty minutes.

Unfortunately, it takes very little energy to create both good and bad effects within the body due to EMWs. Keep in mind that any time an electric current is present, there will be an associated electromagnetic field. Prolonged simultaneous exposure to a low (yet beyond human adaptation) or high gauss strength of both magnetic fields has been observed to be capable of producing POSITIVE magnetic field effects (lethargy, fatigue, illness, and so on) on biological systems.

The Gauss Effect

The EMWs you read about coming off overhead wires, televisions, and microwave ovens, create POSITIVE charges within the body. Their "throw-away" waves are unused energy coming from these devices and are measured by "gauss," their measurement of EMWs (like kilowatts are to electricity).

Named after Carl Friedrich Gauss, the Gauss Meter measures voltage that is produced when a magnetic field crosses an electrical current. If the current remains the same, then a small change in the magnetic field produces a similar and predictable change in the voltage.

The human body can normally take about 1.05–50 gauss a day, but repeated assault of over 50-gauss will interrupt the negative charges from the brain, thus placing the cells into trauma. Amazingly, and unfortunately, there have been reports of electrical pylons over people's homes, emitting 600-gauss of EMWs per day! Computers do not normally create this much energy, but think of the office building with all its steel superstructure. This superstructure becomes a "Faraday Cage" impeding EMWs from flowing through the walls and outside the building. So, the workers are assaulted day after day with minimal doses of EMWs.

In addition to cell erosion, desquamation occurs, leaving the skin feeling dry and tight. The peripheral capillaries become dilated and red. EMWs do create a thermal effect in the body, which, when controlled, can be beneficial, but in the case of capillaries, dead cell build-up and traumatized secretive glands lead to rosacea-like conditions.

Pigmentation Issues

Bad EMWs can adversely affect the pineal gland, the main producer of melanin. In addition, the function of the melanocyte is to rush melanin to the skin's surface when ANY trauma is present. This includes sun damage, squeezing a pimple, or radiation from computers screens.

At the first sign of excess trauma, these little defense cells rush to the skin's surface where they quickly turn brown and try to shield their territory. In as much as the skin is like a landscape full of hills and valleys, the melanin will congregate in various areas unevenly, resulting in hyperpigmentation.

Slow but persistent assault of EMWs will wake up melanin as much as a day at the beach, the same protection (at least 30 SPF daily).

The world is surrounded by magnetic fields generated by the earth, solar storms, changes in the weather and everyday electrical devices. Recently, scientists have discovered that external magnetic fields can affect the body in both positive and negative ways, and the clinical observations are serious eye openers.

Positive Magnetic Fields and their Effects

The following examples of positive magnetic fields that one may experience on a day-to-day basis include:

- Televisions;
- Computers;
- Cell phones;
- Alarm clocks;
- Motors;
- Office equipment;
- Electrical wiring;
- Microwave ovens;
- Electric blankets;
- Power lines;
- Radio and cell phone towers;
- Fluorescent lights;

- Smart Meters; and,
- Wi-Fi.

The frequency at which a magnetic field is pulsed determines whether or not it is harmful. For example, the frequency of the electrical current used in homes in the United States is 60 cycles per second, or hertz (HZ). In contrast, normal frequencies of the human brain during waking hours range from 8 to 22 Hz, while in sleep they can drop to as low as 2 Hz.

The higher frequencies present in artificial electrical currents may disturb the brain's natural resonant frequencies and in time lead to cellular fatigue.

The Physiological Effects of Positive Magnetic Fields

The following are examples of the physiological effects of positive magnetic fields include:
- Produces acid;
- Produces oxygen deficiency;
- Evokes cellular edema;
- Exacerbates existing symptoms;
- Accelerates microorganism replication; speeds up infections;
- Biologically disorganizing;
- Increases pain and inflammation;
- Governs wakefulness and action;
- Evokes catabolic hormone production;
- Produces toxic end products of metabolism;
- Produces free radicals; and,
- Speeds up electrical activity of the brain.

The power and proximity of positive magnetic fields to your energy field are very important, and sources should be investigated with a Gauss meter to understand their frequency. In addition to that, understanding how to "neutralize" these positive magnetic fields becomes very important.

There are fewer places more important to neutralize these frequencies than in an airport or an airplane, for these reasons.

Positive magnetic fields have been associated with cancer, depression, chromosomal abnormalities, inflammation and learning difficulties.

Negative Magnetic Fields and Their Effects

Negative magnetic field therapy has been used effectively in the treatment of:
- Cancer;
- Rheumatoid arthritis;
- Infections and inflammation;
- Headaches and migraines;
- Insomnia and other sleep disorders;
- Circulatory problems;
- Fractures and pain; and,
- Environmental stress, among others.

Understanding the sources of negative and positive magnetic frequencies, and how to avoid and use them effectively, is a key component to an overall wellness plan.

My advice is to identify the worst offenders and avoid them as much as possible, and keep in touch with the earth to discharge them appropriately.

17

Stem Cell Therapy: Myth or Medical Breakthroughs?

Stem cells are now the latest rage globally. Claims of skin rejuvenation using stem cells from plants, animals and even unborn human fetuses (which remain against USA regulations).

In my opinion, out of all the hype and pseudo-science that accompanies the marketing of these products, there is absolutely nothing that remotely resembles the truth!

From the beginning, clever marketers have claimed that cells from the "stems" of plants are the magic factor. While it's true that many beneficial micronutrients can be harvested from plant stems, roots, leaves and fruit, none of them have anything to do with real stem cell activity. In fact, performing a radical resurfacing on the skin via acids or other exfoliants encourages our own stem cell activity as part of the healing mode after injury! But again, this is not real skin regeneration or stimulation of the skin's many cellular functions and structure, only the repair of a breach or irritation at the point of trauma.

Sometimes the claims of stem cells in products are so outrageous and illogical that I wonder how anyone could possibly buy into it. The latest one is the infinite variety of Stem Cell Therapy hoaxes that have abounded for a few years internationally and despite enormous testing and research to the contrary, have flourished.

Plant stem cells, animal stem cells, and even human stem cells can NOT possibly do anything when put into a product, being at that point just dead protein. And, the products that these stem cells are based in already have a plethora of proteins, nutrients, anti-oxidants, and peptides that the skin DOES benefit from, and without the cost hike of the added stem cells.

Plant stem cells, animal stem cells, and even human stem cells can NOT possibly do anything when put into a product, being at that point just dead protein.

Epigenics

Products claiming to "trigger" stem cells in our skins, "Epigenics," is a field of genetics that use external factors that switch genes on and off that affects how cells read the genetic codes outside of the normal DNA sequence. This practice is still what I call the "iffy" stage and not totally proven, although the field is interesting and worth research.

There are thousands of stem cells in our bodies that are at work constantly repairing the damage we go through just by living. All of them are organ-specific but can be "moved around" within the confines of the organ, like moving from one house to another in the same neighborhood. Instead of trying to add bogus cells to the skin, why not work with specific stem cells that live right there in our skin?

At the bottom of the numerous hair follicles (including near-invisible villous facial hairs) is a rich source of baby-stem-cells surrounding the erector pili muscle. Up a little further on the hair shaft itself is "the bulge," another source of new stem cells.

Of course, these are mesoderm and ectoderm cells, the much-touted mesenchymal stem cell is not involved until much further in muscle tissue (some scientists are saying that these may not be stem cells at all). These two groups co-exist to initiate all repairs and growth in the hair follicle.

There are thousands of stem cells in our bodies that are at work constantly repairing the damage we go through just by living.

Langerhans Cells, Keratinocytes and Melanocytes

What if we could expose these stem cells with a special treatment involving a mild trauma? The next step would be to get them past their mitotic response, sort of a rubber band action that occurs when we try to move stem cells "out of their house" into a new house where they can differentiate and evoke massive new repair to the surrounding tissue. In other words, new skin. This could include Langerhans cells, Keratinocytes and Melanocytes! Then the next step would be to move these baby stem cells along the correct genetic pathways or "roads" to the keratinocytes, fibroblasts and all other skin cell functions in the same neighborhood, the epidermis.

I already knew we could perform step one easily (but carefully) and the next steps are already in the works with the help of a team of scientists composed of Dr. Jay Lokhande, a genius at botanical engineering and bio-sciences in medicine, and along with his wife who is a research specialist in gene mapping.

In-vivo Testing

The current protocol in-vivo testing will comprise of a 4-step protocol which begins by opening the channels to the "bulge" and erector pili stem cells. This will be in the form of a special and very delicate pH adjustment formula which opens the door to the epidermis without trauma or injury or by-passing the shunts in the skin with "needling."

There will be rapid cryo-therapy and thermogenics, back and forth to sort of "pull and push" cell groups into memory status followed by a serum mount, and enzymatic occlusion and reverse osmosis application, a final serum mount, and then the appropriate 3-day crème base home regimen and oral capsule designed for collagen matting.

I did present this working hypothesis at a medical conference at Riga, Latvia on November 7th, 2016 to a global group of scientists and physicians. The questions will of course be daunting and the in-vivo testing that will occur before clinical trials.

At DMK International, we already have our focus on a specific group of skin Stem Cells. There will eventually be other stem cell protocols and groups for other parts of the body, but I am focused on the epidermis only. And we do have a base protocol. Finalizing our treatment tools is now in progress. We know that the skin and body are equipped like a superior organic computer, to repair itself.

Our independent Gene Marker Lab tested our compounds in-vivo and discovered an amazing amount of RNA activity, at which point we sighed with relief! At least we knew we were on the right track with viable formulae, and that what remained as the protocols of a portal and a domino effect in the cells. We realized also that there would be many variables in treatment due to age, gender and ethnicity, as well as skin anomalies. How would this "new cell regeneration" affect acne, psoriasis, dermatitis, and other conditions?

Basal cell carcinoma is another issue and mystery to consider. Should these things be removed first? Or, will they be suppressed and indeed removed by the onset of healthy, new tissue?

The clinical trials march on. I truly feel on the tip of a very big iceberg which may include other medical ramifications, such as skin graft procedures, Mons punch grafts, and burn victims. The application is endless.

Stem Cells and Regenerating Skin

Years ago, stem cells and growth factors became hero ingredients in skin care formulations. Some brands have claimed plant-based stem cells helped reproduce human stem cells and growth factors directly changing the behavior of human DNA. Here are a few facts on stem cells in skincare products. Let's start by clearing up some confusion about the roles that stem cells and growth factors performed in regenerating skin, namely human biology versus skincare ingredients: growth factors are proteins that regulate cellular growth, their proliferation and under controlled conditions, maintain healthy skin structure.

Growth factors are secreted by all cell types that make up the epidermis (outer layer of skin) and dermis (the layer of skin between the epidermis and subcutaneous tissue), including keratinocytes, fibroblasts and melanocytes. Growth factors are naturally occurring regulatory molecules. They stimulate cell and tissue function through influencing cell differentiation by changing their biochemical activity.

Regulating the rate of proliferation, certain beta glucans are in this class, enhancing dendrite strength in the Langerhans cells, turning the macrophages at the end of each dendrite into a weapon of mass destruction against free radicals, bacterial attack, viral and even parasitic invasion!

Medical stem cell implantation plays a role as back-up support to the implanted cells and potential auto-immune rejection. So far there have been many successes aspirating fresh stem cells from hip bones and re-injecting them into injured areas such as a torn meniscus. These are mesenchymal stem cells, cells that can develop into distinct mesenchymal tissue such as bone, tendons, muscles, adipose tissue cartilage, nerve tissue, blood and blood cells. However, this is a far cry from crèmes, serums and so on, in skin care.

Do Plant Stem Cells in Skin-Care Products Work?

The most common question that I am asked about stem cells, is how do the plant stem cells in a crème or gel serum work with your own stem cells? The answer is, THEY DON'T.

As a way of inflicting miniature wounds, technicians scratch cultured plant tissue. This damage stimulates the plant's stem cells to react and heal, inducing the formation of new stem cells on the wounded surfaces. After slow replication and division on the outside, new cells fashion a large accumulation of colorless cells, known as callous. Cells composing the callous divide into cells that do not carry the specific features of individuated plant cells. This callous is used as an ingredient in facial crèmes. In fact, it is the pluripotent (human) downstream differentiated plant cells that are the ones that possess the biochemical machinery required to produce the myriad of regenerative activity in the human body, including the skin.

Stem cells that would be included in extracts derived from plants that have pharmaceutical or other value (e.g. quinine, digitalis, aloe Vera, etc.) would not be active, although the other botanical micronutrients may very well be! Think of them as "skin food" not stem cell therapy.

Plant totipotent stem cells do not produce substances capable of affecting other cells. Callouses are forced upon living plant stems to encourage new baby cells, harvested and then put into crèmes as "stem cell therapy." Even rubbing human stem cells on the skin would never work. They must be alive in the product despite any effective delivery mechanism.

Plant stem cells have nothing to do with the human genetic blue print. There has been some argument that these "callouses," or other plant stem cell extracts have many micro nutrients that benefit skin. This is no more true than other aspects of a plant, which includes roots, leaves, buds, flowers and fruit.

A potent botanical offering into skin cells that evoke an ionic transfer, a cellular impact of a physiological change (or I should say, a reverse to homeostasis), depends largely on where the plant is grown, how it is prepared for extraction and how it is processed into a product with bio-availability that is still active—AND the delivery system into the skin.

We should look at which Phyto chemicals that skin cells respond positively to and what they recognize, how we can influence and support growth factors and life cycle of cells. My methods have always been to work with the body's chemistry. Even if plant stem cells DID have a biological energy kick start, research concludes that stem cells are just too large to penetrate the lipid barrier of the epidermis, even if they could be somehow kept alive in a crème, serum etc.

There is hope in stem cell research for total skin revision, however. Keep in mind that every time we do any kind of aggressive exfoliation, we are calling upon stem cells in the healing process. Nevertheless, this is normally not very well controlled or targeted and the healing is spotty or focused on only the areas of the epidermis where trauma is the most virulent. Rebecca James Gadberry's dissertation on Epigenetics pointed this out.

There is hope in stem cell research for total skin revision.

Using our OWN skin stem cells—of which we have a rich supply at any age, although the amount decreases slowly with time—requires the following steps:

1. Getting to them with minimum inflammatory response (although some is needed);
2. Getting the stem cells OUT of their "house" and on a genetic pathway to another "house" in the skin such as a keratinocyte or a fibroblast cell; and,
3. Maintaining the differentiation over a period of 47 days, at least until fresh epidermal tissue is maximized.

There are so many variables, but I thought maybe it could be done. So, I recruited an international team of doctors, botanists and biochemists to take a leap of faith on a project like this with no commercial aspect other than to see if it can be done.

There are many types of stem cells with a variety of special functions. All are Interconnected but organ specific. It is like a large puzzle that is there and has been since the birth of our plant. We are just now finding a few pieces of the puzzle and seeing where they go.

Embryonic Stem Cells and Adult Stem Cells

The two main types of stem cells are embryonic stem cells (ES) and adult stem cells (such as somatic stem cells). Other sub types such as induced pluripotent stem cells (PCS's) are lab produced by re-programming adult cells to express ES characteristics. In skin, tissue specific (or somatic) are more specialized than embryonic stem cells. Typically, these types of stem cells can generate different cell types for the specific tissue or organ in which they live. In short, if you're checking out procedures do your homework.

I encourage you to read all you can and ask the experts and know that you'll find ever-changing knowledge.

It has long been my contention as I look back from now, from my 75th year, that the cells of the body are not programmed to die easily. They are programmed to stay alive if possible, given the right maintenance and environmental surroundings.

The StemZyme Protocol

At DMK International, we have completed our required male and female test trials with what we now call The StemZyme Protocol. I am a bit awed by the fact that up until now, no one has ever done this before!

I owe a great deal to my colleague, Dr. Jayant Lokahnde, MD., a brilliant young bio-engineer trained in Ayurveda herbology by Masters in India.

Without his research into how to enter genomic pathways to other cells in the epidermis—after getting hair follicle baby stem cells past mitotic shock—and place them in regenerative areas such as keratinocytes, Langerhans, melasmasomes, fibroblast, and so on, I could never have realized the potential of this remarkable process that takes 50 days total—after initial "gateway" opening treatment.

We will medically publish because outside of the obvious age management benefits of stronger, more turgid and plumped appearing skin, I see a definite role StemZyme may be able to play in tissue transplantation and burn victims, including radiation in oncology treatment.

I see the applications as endless.

18

Bacteria in a Bottle

The human body, including the topical layer, the skin, is host to thousands of bacterial and fungal species, some of which are harmful, and some known to be beneficial.

The skin flora is different to that of the gut, although a stomach that is suffering from bacterial overload, **Leaky Gut Syndrome** or other intestinal disorders can be reflected in skin health, as well. This is especially true in cases of acne, rosacea and other dermatological disorders.

Microbiome

We have already maintained the healthy microbiome of the skin for decades with Enzyme treatments, fractionated oils resembling sebum, and an herb water blend to replicate the acid mantle along with Beta glucans. Lactic acid that have also been playing a role in microbiota maintenance.

The professional therapy field has not totally ignored the skin microbiota, but until recently no one had identified this huge iceberg in our physiognomy with a name. Rebecca James Gadberry did a comprehensive lecture on skin microbiome back in 2015 but suddenly, this year it's on everyone's lips!

Microbiome is yet another trending buzz word with a plethora of creams claiming to restore the microbiome to the skin. I have researched a few of these and sadly found out it was mostly dried yogurt in a cream with a lot of other things, not bad, but it had nothing to do with skin microbiome.

If the manufacturer understands the real concept behind skin micro-flora, I can envision some of these newly developed products having true potential. Let's start with a basic analysis of the skins natural friendly bacteria, most in the gram positive category. Gram-positive, or negative, refers to a categorizing, or identifying, bacteria.

Natural Friendly Bacteria

Chemoorganotrophs: Organisms that produce energy from organic material and converts into other natural materials that open the door to extracellular enzymes. This can include dead skin cells and organic debris collected on the epidermis.

Pre-Biotics: Can fire up the friendly microbiome colonies located in the for mentioned areas and the reduction of dead keratinocytes. This will allow the healthy bacteria to scatter across the skin killing off unfriendly (gram negative) bacterial overloads.

Pro-Biotics: The end product of bacteria in the microbiome which can include many compounds already used in skincare such as lactic acid. They also help maintain the colonies while warding off further attack of unfriendly bacteria and fungus.
This basic microbiome group is present on healthy skin but acts differently than the same group in our guts.

Actinobacteria: Gram positive—also found in soil, plant decomposition and humus (which may explain why children who get to play in soil often have healthier immune systems).

Bacteroides Fragilis: Normal flora found in the colon, and needed at some level as gram negative for flora balance but can cause infection if overloaded on surrounding tissue in the blood field (micro needling, blading) post-surgery, dermatitis, acne and eczema).

Firmicutes: This gram-negative bacteria can be a major part of bacterial homeostasis, anti-inflammatory and antibiotic.

Proteobacteria: An ultimate predator of gram negative bacteria, capable of acquiring cell nutrients that are present or toxic debris (through nitrogen phagocytosis). This one is a double-edged sword that has to be carefully formulated.

Non-Friendly Bacteria (the Bad Guys)

Micrococci: Not common but can be found on people with poor skin habits and contamination—such as contact dermatitis.

Streptococci: Very bad, not found on normal skin. Lipids are lethal to this group—such as healthy sebum or a fractioned oil resembling sebum (few oils are "comedogenic" as popularly believed). Micrococci is symbiotic to virus such as herpes and can start in the mouth and spread to the skin and then to another person.

Malassezia: Fungi naturally found on skin and sometimes mis-diagnosed as eczema, can cause hypo and hyperpigmentation.

One of my field educators applied one of my samples on a male of Asian descent who suffered from hyperpigmented eczema for several years. All symptoms vanished in 48 hours! He had Malessezia.

THE SUPER STARS!

Lactobacillus: Found in fermented foods, limits the amounts of parthenogenic bacteria, parasites (rosacea-causing Demodex mites) and virus spread.

Bifidobacterium: Found in "functional foods," promotes probiotic activities, and protects against pathogens.

I gained a huge respect for professionals in the field of micro-biology and bacteria, as I contacted colleagues all over the world when it became clear this would be a trend.

I think, like true stem cell research for skin, that we are on the tip of a very large iceberg here—that if approached properly, without rushing to get products out to capitalize on popular trends, will benefit many people. This may change a large section of the skincare industry in the skin disease arena—non-medically.

To avoid intervention from regulatory government departments here and abroad, we must always refer to helping the skin heal itself by providing the maximum care and environment.

I maintain that any results-driven products should be used only for skin conditions that are deficit in normal microbiome. But the real story is when trends starts, everybody wants to try it! Nothing wrong with that—but products addressing this are not that easy to compound. Living spores must be kept inert in a container until used.

We have successfully done this—a very tedious and bothersome process in the lab. Relief has been reported in many cases of face and body disorders that never seemed to go away and were often misdiagnosed as eczema or "contact dermatitis."

Skin Microbiome

New research into the mysteries of Eczema and other inflammatory dermatitis, where the microbiome is out of homeostasis, has lead me to explore better and more efficient ways to proliferate and maintain the skin's microbiome at levels to ward off the invasive "bad" bacteria, while simultaneously protecting the epidermis with beneficial bacteria.

Prebiotics

Prebiotics also help convert detoxified waste materials, hydrolyzed proteins, into active proteins or "skin food." These are known under the name CHEMOORGANOTROPHS—which are capable of breaking down organic material, such as redundant dead skin cells, and convert them into organic material. This opens the door to kick-starting dormant (often due to age) extracellular enzymes—particularly the transferase gang whose job is to send "wake up" messages across cell membranes, telling them to get to work again!

Skin Bacteria: the Good, the Bad and the Ugly

At a conference I attended, one speaker referred to skin bacteria as "the Good, the Bad and the Ugly" (from the old spaghetti western starring Clint Eastwood). In a way, his analogy was spot on. Our skins are colonized by basically good bacteria that make up the defense mechanisms designed to ward off attack by the bad guys who wreak havoc with the repair tools that we are all born with.

The "ugly" would be the parasites we all possess; look at a blown-up photo on Google of the Demodex mite, one of the culprits in Rosacea! Nothing more nightmare-ish ugly then those little varmints!

Let's identify the unmutated bacteria to better understand what we as skin practitioners are up against.

Bacteroides Fragilis. These species are part of the normal flora found in the human colon. Generally commensal but CAN cause infection if let into the blood stream via micro needling or PRP on the skin or on surrounding tissue following surgery. They can become "bad" during trauma from acne, dermatitis, rosacea and eczema.

Firmicutes. These Gram-positive bacteria with very strong cell walls does have some species of lactobacillus—the good guys. They act as a major portion of bacterial homeostasis (the most important word in microbiome) and are anti-inflammatory and antibiotic.

Conversely Gram negative bacilli makes up a very small portion of the skin flora, and are mainly found in toe webs and Axilla. They are the P.U factor from armpits. We do need them to create homeostasis in the entire skin flora.

Proteobacteria. This strain can create nitrogen phagocytosis, meaning the acquisition of both toxic debris AND cell nutrients. However, they can be strong predators of bad bacteria that is gram negative.

Lactobacillus Plantarium. We get these beneficial bacteria when we eat fermented foods such a sauerkraut or Kim Chi. To suggest as "sauerkraut mask" may not be so outrageous after all!

S. Epidermis and S. Aureus. These two hate one another and are most found in eczema and Atrophic Dermatitis research.

S. Epidermis is a major denizen of skin and in some areas make up more than 90% of aerobic flora! This could partially explain why tribes of people in remote South American villages, wearing few garments and living practically out in the open and possess no commercial antibiotic products, have almost no history of skin disorders. Interestingly, even teens in these tribes do not get acne.

I learned this from an old American Indian Shaman many years ago, when I was researching natural surfactants indigenous to the North American continent. He showed me the bark from the White Oak tree and the rhizome from the Century Cactus and how it was pounded, pulped and mixed with water to cleanse body, hair and even teeth. "No pimples on my people—ever," he claimed.

S. Aureus, on the other hand is a bad guy, very common on the nose and perineum and accounts for 40% in normal adults, but this can rise to 80-100% on the skin of patients with various skin disorders such as Atopic Dermatitis.

S, Epidermis can roll right over S. Aureus, and destroy it in minutes.

Malassezia. This is in the fungus category and is natural to almost everyone's skin. When allowed to become predominant, sometimes accompanying eczema, it can cause both hypo and hyperpigmentation, thus many times mis-diagnosed.

Pre and Pro Biotics can help set up defenses against this little devil, but primary enzymatic removal treatment is required to get rid of it with ongoing Pre and Post biotic home treatment to maintain homeostasis. Older cases can vanish within 48 after treatment.

Other possible bacteria include:

Micrococci. Not common but frequently found on normal skin that reflects poor skin habits, diet and contaminated surroundings.

Streptococci. This very bad actor is not seen on normal skins. Lipids such as healthy sebum are lethal to this species. Some of these species start in the mouth and then spread to the skin—very symbiotic to virus such as herpes. In fact, virus, bacteria and parasites love to party together leading to many flawed diagnoses and "causes" of dozens of skin disorders such as "Acne Rosacea"—used for decades until the medical field disowned it as a disease. I still hear it used globally by dermatologists.

Bifidobacterium. These are the angels of bacteriology and most often used in "functional foods" and supplements due to their health promoting probiotic properties, and act as protection, not predators against pathogens.

So much about the micro biotic world is yet unknown. Many of us through trial and error, have tried things outside of acceptable medical practice and unknowingly been headed in the right direction.

The more we learn about the microbiome, the more we will understand that it is not the presence of bacteria that causes all the anomalies of skin disorders but rather, the imbalance of the types of bacteria that live on our skins.

One outstanding imbalance right under our noses all along was the large amounts of S. Aureus that is always present in Eczema cases. One theory was that S. Aureus was causing the dry, itchy and inflamed symptoms of the disease. To fight these researchers applied copious amount of pure Epidermis and S. hominis over the affected area (via cultures in a petri dish). The bad guys died within seconds. Follow up treatment by infusing the good bacteria in a topical crème on a human subject and dropped the eczema by 90% in minutes.

Lysates

The use of Lysates also looks promising. Cell lysis is a purifying process used in laboratories to break open cells to purify and study their contents. Enzymes, detergents of chaotropic agents may be used in this process.

Lysis is also used for DNA/RNA extraction and protein purification. It can also be used as "mulch" to help grow friendly bacteria. Lysates are also powerful inducers of specific immune response against bacterial infections, especially pulmonary. At the moment, we don't fully understood why.

Using Bacteria to Fight Skin Conditions

Other global studies are researching which bacteria will fight specific skin conditions. One discovered that Lactobacillus plantarum lotion reduced skin redness and pustule size in persons with acne vulgaris. Others still are investigating ammonia-oxidizing bacteria. This bacteria metabolizes ammonia, a major component of sweat. Bacteria that metabolizes ammonia may someday be used for acne treatment and even chronic wounds, such as osteomyelitis.

For these studies, a strain of Nitrosomonas eutropha, isolated from soil in double blind tests, resulted in incredibly improved skin on scalps and faces.

This brought to mind one of my trips to Indonesia where I saw naked children living in what we would consider filthy or unclean conditions.

I noted the kids had amazing skin, good muscle tone and

white teeth, yet they were swimming in canals of unsanitary brown water with debris. Apparently their immune systems had grown to tolerate what became a friendly bacteria, a favorable skin microbiota. Basically, this is nitric oxide which dilate the blood vessels making it easier for the heart to pump blood flow through the body. Nitric oxide also helps regulate inflammation.

The more we learn about bacteria, the more we see that the days of trying to heal skin diseases by destroying bacteria on the skin may be over sooner than later, and, outside FDA and EU regulations.

It will be certain that our professional tools will include spraying or petrissage bacteria over our clients faces and teaching them to be less antibacterial conscious (outside of washing our hands several times a day).

Bacterial diversity will become a buzz word and hopefully a trend.

Trends are only stable however, when the trend evolves into effective concepts in science that not only change the way we think—but what we do in our practice.

The field of bacteriology is at an infancy stage. As we research, we learn to use common sense on how the chemistry of the body really works, not just how we imagine it should work. This will allow us to put together practical concepts that professional wellness practitioners, and clients alike, can use.

Here are some other things we are learning about:

Pre-Biotics:

- Stimulate dying, but still viable, bacteria on less than healthy skin;

- Induce the detoxifying waste recycling process, rendering it as autophagy which converts inactive proteins into acting proteins necessary as "skin cell food" while supporting the skins natural skin repair modalities;

- Help boost Langerhans and other skin immune defenses; and,

- Calms and repress inflammatory conditions.

Post and Probiotics:

- Maintains the Probiotic bifudo cultures;

- Helps to maintain active skin nutrients applied after application;

- Increases metabolic activity of skin cells and immune systems;

- Protects against environmental stress including solar damage and pollution;

- Protects against overload of bad bacteria, which takes healthy skin out of homeostasis; and,

- Is helpful in cases of glycation.

The field of Probiotic is new, and a great many of products I have seen so far are akin to dried yogurt in a crème. I can only say that all the above be present in the products, and, the culture's must be alive.

My DMK International project (which I call Enbioment), has addressed the re-establishment of the microbiome film which has shown remarkable, often seemingly "over-night," alleviation of eczema, a skin fungus often misdiagnosed as hyper (brown) or hypo (white) pigmentation.

We have learned to control a vast organism that controls our immune system. This small step will prove to change the entire skin industry as well. As always, keep checking the DMK website for updates in this interesting and ever-changing field of skin care, and skin revision.

19

INSIDE OUT: Holistic Wellness and Lifestyle Monitoring

The word "holistic" has again become a popular buzz word. It seems to refer to an "all-natural," "organic" or non-medical intervention to all the illness and diseases we suffer, including aging.

I never bought into this trend. I prefer to think that what my global team and I do is "holistic" because we look at the human body as connected with each function related to the next.

The word "holistic" has been around as long as I have and that is seven-plus decades! In the 1960s the word was bandied about by so-called practitioners in tie-dyed robes reeking of patchouli oil, who would wave their crystals up and down the front of your body while chanting, claiming they were cleansing you of toxins. They would offer "homemade" herbal products titled under "holistic medicine," much of which would grow a fine layer of mold after a couple of weeks due to the absence of "cancer causing" preservative!

For these reasons, when I would hear myself described as a "holistic scientist," I would feel vaguely annoyed at this title. I've been called "revolutionary" by the Swedish press, as described with hilarity in my book *The Maybelline Prince*—the story of my relationships over time in connection with the Maybelline company, principally with the founder's sister-in-law, Evelyn (both pre and after days and then my subsequent founding of my own skin-care dynasty, DMK International).

By modern definitions, I would privately spell the word "wholistic" because it encompasses everything, rather than focusing on or treating one symptom in one area at a time. My Research and Development lab has just enough equipment to process a formula into a usable tool, but the formulations are based upon what the body requires for the healing process, or what revision of tissue was needed to take place. In this case, I am looking at the WHOLE picture, primarily the root cause of the disorder that needs to be treated, in addition to its symptoms and appearance.

For many decades I have been a holistic practitioner, teacher and Guru, per se. In truth, there is no single miracle ingredient that is a cure-all. When diagnosing the skin, it's important to understand that everything is symbiotic and connected. The knee bone really is connected to the thigh bone. Structure, as well as functionality, is a vital part of everyone's skin.

> There is no single miracle ingredient that is a cure-all.

What is "Wellness"?

The Wikipedia definition of wellness is "alternative medicine" and "freedom from illness." Both descriptors fit, but in our field of addressing skin, I like to think of wellness as "preventative" treatments and home use regimens.

In the US there has been widespread popularity amongst the age 9 to 13-year-old crowd for using products designed to protect their delicate skins before solar damage does its insidious permanent damage on the DNA of their little cells (and before the pizza wagon of acne smacks them in their faces)! These young people are learning about what keeps a skin cell healthy and what the mitochondria does, as well as what too-long in the sun does with its heating up a free radical soup in their tender tissues called lipofuscin.

Wellness also has to do with diet and nutrition. As always, avoid using products that do not really work or could create contraindications. As I always say, "Think of your cells as a little walled city with a King and Two Queens living in a castle in the center, surrounded by warehouses that store the foods they need, and, a power station that keeps everything going."

I just described the functions of a skin cell.

An Inside Out Approach

One of the things that I am impressed about in Australia is the availability of tests that therapists can order for their clients, whether it be sputum, feces, urine or saliva. The results of these tests don't give them the right to diagnose any illness or prescribe medications, like an MD, but it can give them a better insight as to why the skin is suffering severe anomalies. This thorough approach helps a skin-care specialist adjust the topical treatment protocol according to what is needed, and issue the right home products.

It also helps determine if the client would benefit from being referred to other practitioners licensed for disease treatment, or could benefit from specialized care.

This trend is becoming more popular in the USA mainly because wellness centers are becoming more popular than the trendy "Medi Spa." My company, DMK International, is working with a group in Mexico who have built 150 Time-Share condominiums where people undergoing complete wellness programs can stay. This will include IV vitamin drips, Chelation, Plasma Return during surgery (a forerunner of the popular "vampire face life"), adipose fat reassignment, nutrition and weight loss altered lifestyle programs, and more. I already have my yearly live cell therapy injections there, which saves me an expensive trip to Nassau in the Bahamas where I used to go since 1984! The point is, more and more, people seek wellness, prevention, and anti-aging treatments. And, they seek these wholistic treatments, and in places designed with their good health in mind.

As I earlier explained, more people want to look good, and, feel good. The body DOES change inside and out as we age. At a certain point, stomach ailments, joint pains, and a plethora of baddies that were previously unnoticed during the earlier years suddenly out-weigh vanity! Preventative wellness is the key to ALL these things, and I am thankful I unwittingly practiced it all these decades, starting with a health conscious and forward-thinking Mother.

Lifestyle Monitoring

As baby boomers abound by living longer, lifestyles are altered. People want to look good and at every age. But just having treatments or plastic surgery done, is not going to suddenly "turn back time," as Cher sings in her legendary song. Speaking of Cher, she is one of the most genuine and hard-working women I've had the pleasure to meet. For some time, I had created a special skin foundation just for her (not for sale). When I met her, I found a warm, feminine woman whose appearance defied her years. Most impressive was that her attitude is timeless, and ageless.

Life-style monitoring is the thing, now. There are many Lifeline therapists who counsel their clients with the Lifeline life-style monitoring techniques. These cover a broad range of illnesses and even psychological problems that exacerbate acne and other skin disorders.

Years ago, in my first Chicago clinic, I established a regimen for weight loss that was a Life Style Monitoring system. Each patient who came to me and my partner, Dr. Augustine, filled out a lengthy life-style questionnaire that covered health and dietary habits, food cravings, physical activities, medical history, medications, and so on. Using this and blood-work, we then tailored a food plan prescribing appropriate supplements, and with good results. Even better, was that our clients experienced fewer cravings, and lost weight.

Holistic wellness, lifestyle monitoring—all are trends overlapping in concept. Many more people today are growing self-aware and realize that they can be healthy and "well," and that the quality of this self-care is a reflection of their health, beginning in the appearance of their skin.

20

Trends in Skin Health

I have been very honored to have some of the finest physicians and medical research men and women on my team over the years. As a senior statesman now, these incredible folks have given me almost guru status, yet it is their work in the field in many countries has enabled us to achieve results in cases where a patient has such horrendous skin anomalies or life changing traumas that they had lost all hope of appearing and feeling normal. I am privileged to participate in such changes throughout the world and build in the best practices into my practice and my world-wide affiliates. Skin care is an ever-important field: the recent medical trends of injectables offers quick fixes but are not permanent, and many times fail if the patient has skin starving for nutrients or literally breaking down from years of abuse.

For fifty years I have been involved in that "gray area" of the medical and aesthetic word. It was very disheartening to see incredible results happening with topical skin revision treatments and yet not be able to make any claims that would border on the sanctified area of medical.

In the last three decades many physicians attached their names and MD's to skincare ranges under the belief that the customers would somehow believe that the products were "better" and "medically based," but the facts are, there are basic category products that can be sold or prescribed under medical or cosmetic regulations.

The term "cosmeceuticals" has been tossed around as some sort of descriptive category, but it's not legally recognized by the FDA.

During the past decade of my global travel participating in medical and aesthetics conferences, I witnessed the trends of the aesthetician performing protocols that maximizes skin health, better immune defense against permanent damage or scars, and longer lasting effects from the new age of fillers and "re-dis-solvable" threads.

I myself have viewed some stunning innovations! As an example, I had spoken at a medical conference in Russia, and sat in as Dr. Sabine Zenker was lecturing on the new generation of fillers, displaying her remarkable "face mapping" techniques.

Based on the theory that healthy skin holds fillers in place longer (unhealthy skin perceives the hyaluronic base of fillers as a nutrient and gobbles it up fast), Dr. Zenker marked the clients face with a surgeon's pen into different levels, then proceeded to use multiple syringes with various bore sizes and different viscosity sod fillers to inject in multiple levels of the sub epidermis and epidermis. I watched in awe as she layered "pearls" of filler along bone areas in the face and neck and worked her way upwards, switching fillers and inserting the syringe at angles I had never thought possible.

The results were remarkable!

Dissolvable Sutures, Enzyme Masks

Dr. Alexander, from our Moscow Research Center, also displayed his latest innovation of facelift threads. The problem with previous "feather lift" sutures is that they all retracted quickly, often forming coiled granulomas under the skin, and at times even surfaced as lumps or bumps that had to be surgically removed.

Dr. Alexander's method, however, was to apply a series of skin tightening enzyme treatments to strengthen the epidermis and flush out toxins and other effluvia, leaving behind a skin with good circulation and natural epidermal growth factors. He then inserted dissolvable sutures under the epidermis in vertical formations, and in corner of the nasal labial folds up to the pre-auricular area. Once the sutures were placed, his therapist applied an enzyme masque that works on the reverse osmosis principle, dilating the capillaries of the skin and increasing circulation around the sutures.

After six weeks the sutures dissolve and precise adhesions with new collagen are formed in definite skin tightening pathways, as opposed to the general "hit and miss" collagen-forcing modalities brought on by various machines that have been so popular.

We know the mechanism of creating trauma under the skin to force new collagen, and there are many machines using thermal energy or intense light laser that achieves this. In my opinion, the more precise in location with trauma-on-purpose, combined with proper skin revision treatments to reduce inflammation and encourage natural epidermal growth, makes sense.

Like I said, it's happening globally and will change our industry as we know it. You'll have to decide for yourself is you wish to experience the results.

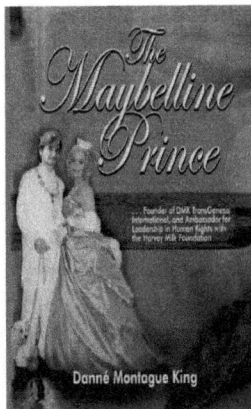

The Maybelline Prince
by Danné Montague-King

The 1970s were known as the era of "sex, drugs & rock 'n' roll." In the midst of all this appeared a woman who had turned the head of Al Capone, married into the famous Maybelline company, and possessed more than enough beauty, magnetism and allure to make men do most anything.

When Evelyn F. Williams and her enigmatic young male companion arrived in Hot Springs, Arkansas, they took over the famous town in a whirlwind of lights, rock 'n' roll, cameras, beautiful people and a grand lifestyle. They created a media frenzy wherever they went and changed people's lives for the better—until the mystery of the Maybelline Queen's fiery death, which some still call an unsolved murder.

This is the uncut version of that high-living time written by the young man who lived it with Evelyn—the man who was supposed to "never be heard from again"—Danné Montague-King, a.k.a., "The Maybelline Prince"—who went on to found a skincare dynasty of his own. Hobnobbing with decadent bluebloods, politicians, movie stars and social activists, Danné amassed a large and loyal following the world over.

Print ISBN: 978-1-940784-14-4 · Digital ISBN: 978-1-940784-15-1

REVIEWS

"Danné King is one of the most dashing, dramatic and accomplished gentlemen I have met in my career as a Hollywood Reporter! You will become fascinated with this man of a thousand faces, and love them all! An exciting tale of love, desire, envy and intrigue.
—Marci Weiner, Entertainment Reporter & Columnist

"This is an exciting, outrageous read—you will like it!"
—Grace Robbins, author of *Cinderella and The Carpetbagger*

"Glorious writing! An exciting book told with tongue-in-

cheek humor and filled with history of a most amazing life and times!"
—Melissa McCarty, Host, Larry King's ORA TV, author of News Girls Don't Cry

"In this breathtakingly honest biography, Danné Montague-King not only lets us in on all the gossip of an extraordinary life well-lived, but also into his soul. It is a roller-coaster ride of emotions, from the hysterically funny to the heart-wrenching—all told by a man with a razor sharp observation and a deep compassion for humanity."
—Frank Howsen, Award-winning Director, Writer & Lyricist

"LIGHTS, CAMERA, ACTION: the modeling gigs, the rock bands, the bodyguards, the fast cars, I was there! Who would not feel like a star, we were the beautiful people, and the spotlight never dimmed. Anyone who passed through 212 Brown Drive left a different person. Danné is a dream maker. Anyone who is fortunate enough to meet Danné would never be the same; it is all a life changing experience! He changed Evelyn's life as well, and 'Miss Maybelline' was never happier!"
—Robert Shannon, Artist, San Miguel, Mexico

"Danné... the king of skin care is now an author. This book tells it like it is and pulls no punches. I was taken aback by a lot of it. The twists and turns and the suspense is mind stimulating. I give it a thumbs up."
—Ron Russell, Television Talk Show Host/Actor

"What an amazing book. "
—Sheena Metal, Talk LA Radio Host